PALEO D_ _ _
COOKBOOK

Choosing the Foods Which Your Ancestors Used to Eat and Get Healthy

(Easy to Prepare Healthy Crock Pot Paleo Recipes)

Melissa Anderson

Published by Tomas Edwards

© **Melissa Anderson**

All Rights Reserved

Paleo Diet Cookbook: Choosing the Foods Which Your Ancestors Used to Eat and Get Healthy (Easy to Prepare Healthy Crock Pot Paleo Recipes)

ISBN 978-1-989744-67-3

All rights reserved. No part of this guide may be reproduced in any form without permission in writing from the publisher except in the case of brief quotations embodied in critical articles or reviews.

Legal & Disclaimer

The information contained in this book is not designed to replace or take the place of any form of medicine or professional medical advice. The information in this book has been provided for educational and entertainment purposes only.

The information contained in this book has been compiled from sources deemed reliable, and it is accurate to the best of the Author's knowledge; however, the Author cannot guarantee its accuracy and validity and cannot be held liable for any errors or omissions. Changes are periodically made to this book. You must consult your doctor or get professional medical advice before using any of the suggested remedies, techniques, or information in this book.

Table of contents

PART 1 1

CHAPTER 1: PALEO DIET 101 2

CHAPTER 2: EAT FOOD, NOT NUTRIENTS 14

CHAPTER 3: THE QUALITY OF YOUR PROTEINS 19

CHAPTER 4: IS MEAT REALLY THAT BAD? 25

CHAPTER 5: PALEO DIET VS DETOX DIET 32

CHAPTER 6: WHY YOU ARE NOT LOSING WEIGHT WITH THE PALEO DIET ... 41

CHAPTER 7: THE IMPORTANCE OF NATURAL FOODS 46

CHAPTER 8: PALEO DIET AFTER THE HOLIDAYS 49

CHAPTER 9: THE IMPORTANCE OF MICRONUTRIENTS 53

CHAPTER 10: THE BEST PALEO FOOD – POMEGRANATE 61

CHAPTER 11: THE PROBLEM WITH NUTRITIONAL STUDIES 66

CHAPTER 12: ANOTHER GREAT PALEO FOOD – KIWI 71

CHAPTER 13: IS LOW CARB A GOOD ALTERNATIVE TO THE PALEO DIET? ... 78

CHAPTER 14: 15 PALEO RECIPES 84

   1. KETOGENIC PANCAKES 84
   2. KETOGENIC MEATBALLS 85
   3. SPICY SCRAMBLED EGGS 86
   4. KETOGENIC BISCUITS 86
   5. VEGETABLE PASSION 87
   6. KETO CURRY 89
   7. KETOGENIC PASTA 89
   8. EGGS AND TUNA 90
   9. AUTUMN TASTES 91
   10. TASTE OF THE SEA 92
   11. CHICKEN AND AVOCADO 93
   12. COCOA AND MINT – A KETO DESSERT 94

13. RICE AND VEGETABLES 95
14. KETOGENIC BRIOCHE 96
15. RICOTTA EXPLOSION 97
1. CHOCOLATE CHIP COCONUT FLOUR COOKIES 97
2. PERFECT PALEO CHOCOLATE CHIP COOKIES 98
3. CROCK POT PALEO COOKIES WITH CHOCOLATE CHIPS 100
4. FARMER BOYS DELIGHT PALEO COOKIE 101
5. CHEWY GRAIN FREE SNICKERDOODLES 102
6. CARROT CAKE CAVEMAN COOKIES 103
7. AVOCADO BANANA COOKIES 104
8. HUGE PALEO COOKIE FOR ONE PERSON 105
9. SOFT & CHEWY DOUBLE CHOCOLATE COOKIES 106
10. PALEO HAZELNUT COOKIES 107
11. PALEO PUMPKIN SPICE CHOCOLATE CHIP COOKIES 108
12. PROBABLY THE HEALTHIEST COOKIES IN THE WORLD. 109
13. PALEO TOFFEE BAR RECIPE 110
14. FLOURLESS MEXICAN HOT CHOCOLATE BROWNIE COOKIES 111
15. PALEO MACADAMIA CRANBERRY COOKIES 113
16. PALEO GINGERSNAP COOKIES 114
17. FLOURLESS CASHEW BUTTER CHOCOLATE CHIP COOKIES 116
18. SKINNY CHOCOLATE PEANUT BUTTER NO BAKE COOKIES 117
19. PEPPERMINT CHOCOLATE CRINKLE COOKIES 118
20. ORANGE BLOSSOM COOKIES 119
21. MAPLE BACON CHOCOLATE CHIP COOKIES 120

CONCLUSION 122

PART 2 123

INTRODUCTION 124

CHAPTER ONE 125

EATING, DIET, AND NUTRITION TO HEALTHY LIVING 125

CHAPTER TWO 131

WHY PALEO DIET? 131

CHAPTER THREE 135

THE ORIGIN OF THE PALEO DIET 135

CHAPTER FOUR 140

ADVANTAGES AND DISADVANTAGES OF THE PALEO DIET........................ 140

CHAPTER FIVE 146

FOODS AND COMMON MISTAKES YOU MUST NOT CONSIDER WHEN ON THE PALEO DIET 146

CHAPTER SIX 160

AMAZING WAYS TO INCORPORATE THE PALEO DIET INTO YOUR LIFESTYLE 160

CHAPTER SEVEN 165

TIME TO PREPARE YOUR KITCHEN FOR THE PALEO DIET 165

CHAPTER EIGHT.. 174

PALEO DIET FOR FAMILIES WITH KIDS 174

CHAPTER NINE 178

PALEO DIET: THE PERFECT BREAKFAST IDEAS.. 178

CHAPTER TEN 184

DAY TO DAY PALEO DIET RECIPES.. 184

CHAPTER ELEVEN 189

SALT AND THE PALEO DIET 189

Part 1

Chapter 1: Paleo Diet 101

The Paleo Diet is a very special diet that has gained considerable popularity, especially in certain environments, in recent years. The basic objective is to return to a style of feeding similar to that of our predecessors hunter-gatherers, a style for which our body would be better adapted and that should allow to eliminate many of the problems related to modernity.
The first to talk about paleo diet was S. Boyd Eaton in a 1985 article titled Paleolithic Nutrition. In this work it was pointed out how the genus Homo, to which we belong, has evolved essentially as a hunter-gatherer, eating meat, that of the prey that could catch, fish, vegetables, fruit seeds, tubers. No legumes, no cereals, no milk, products that have become part of the human diet since just over 10,000 years ago and for which our organism would not yet be adapted. And the transition to a diet based on agricultural products, according to Eaton, would have caused the appearance of a series of problems related to the consumption of foods for which we are fundamentally maladapted. Eaton also examined the diet of the few surviving groups of hunter-gatherers, scattered tribes that mostly survive in inhospitable and marginal environments, from the Kung of the Kalahari to the Hadza of Tanzania, to the Australian aborigines, more or less rich in meat and fish. but without the typical products of sedentary agriculture, to our current diet, to the truth to the tremendous diet of American friends, rich in refined cereals, fats and sodium, underlining how it could be the consumption of "modern" foods at the root of pathologies constantly growing like diabetes, cardiovascular disease, cancer.

A few years later, Staffan Lindeberg, a Swedish doctor, in his Food and Western Disease increased the dose: based his studies on the inhabitants of Kitava Island in New Guinea, whose diet is based on tubers, fruit, coconut and fish, and whose health appears decidedly superior to that of the western average, Lindeberg pointed out that the foods we currently consume in large quantities are foods for which our body is poorly adapted, while the consumption of "ancestral" food would be the basis of the health of iron of the Kitavani. Lindeberg carefully weighed the data, which was in truth, related to the diet of our ancestors and then proceeded to examine the diseases of "modernity" in the light of the data collected, highlighting the important role that, in his opinion, the foods brought to the table from the passage to agriculture they would have played. Lindeberg therefore suggested a diet based on food of vegetable origin, meat, fish, seeds and tubers with the elimination of cereals, legumes and milk, without forgetting to underline also the potential problems related to paleolithic diet.

In 2002 the book The PaleoDiet of the American physiologist Loren Cordain came out, based on his numerous studies on the subject, he went back to underlining how the current diet is essentially "wrong" from the evolutionary point of view, being too recent: the human organism it would not have had materially the time necessary to adapt to the foods fruit of agriculture, foods to avoid in favor of meat and vegetables in quantity.

In these works we try to reason in the field of evolutionary biology, with the aim of finding a rational able to explain the progressive increase of cardiovascular diseases, diabetes, cancer, degenerative and autoimmune diseases, so common in industrialized countries. Both authors point out that for most of the evolutionary history of mankind the diet was based on a few products, available through hunting and gathering. For the distant frugivorous ancestors, the foods of choice were mainly fruits and seeds, but over the course of two million years the various species of the genus Homo have adapted to the consumption of new foods, especially meat, fish in coastal areas, fruit, vegetables , seeds and tubers. The domestication of cereals, legumes and the first animals, which allowed the transition to an agricultural society, was, for our experts, a real disgrace: too recent, from 20,000 to 10,000 years ago, and too rapid for allow the species to adapt adequately. This has resulted in catastrophic consequences: reduced average height, skeletal and dental problems, almost endemic spread of diseases such as diabetes and cardiovascular diseases. A suggestive hypothesis that, however, as we shall see, presents several weak points.

The problem with the paleodieta is what happened next: on the wave of the carbohydrate phobia that grew up in the United States in the last decade, on the paleo wagon skipped subjects of all kinds, especially those related to particular sports environments, proposing variations in which there were industrial quantities of meat, fat at will and above all the inevitable bacon - a kind of bacon that clearly in the Paleolithic era was to be the main food of our hunting friends. All accompanied by the strict exclusion exclusion of cereals, legumes, milk and a plethora of other foods chosen based on tastes and idiosyncrasies of the subject who proposed his personal interpretation of the diet. A saraband that has unfortunately distorted and made a grotesque proposal that was not to be neglected, a confusion that eventually led to stamp the paleo diet as a fad diet, a trendy diet without scientific fundamentals. Fortunately, in recent years there have been many studies that have examined the effects of the paleo diet on various diseases with very interesting results.

Understanding what and how to eat in a paleo diet is not easy: our ancestors who hunted in the savannah unfortunately did not leave us recipe books and the data we have are based on the collection and examination of the waste of ancient settlements, on relative deductions to the anatomical characteristics modified during the evolution, on the analysis of the diet of the few hunter-gatherer populations left in some remote corner of the planet.

The current consensus provides that a paleo diet is based on the consumption of these foods:

Meat
Evolutionary biology studies agree that the consumption of meat, a very nutritionally nutritious food, has been crucial for the evolution of mankind. Obviously our ancestors certainly did not eat hamburgers or breaded chicken medallions. The meat consumed was that of wild animals, lean and with a composition of fatty acids decidedly different from that of today's breeding specimens, with a high presence of stearic acid - which does not cause an increase in cholesterol - high presence of high-quality omega 3 and reduced presence of omega 6, potentially pro-inflammatory if in excess. So we suggest the consumption of meat from animals reared outdoors, with fodder -grass feed is the term for the most performing among you- and not with grains or worse feeds, game and wild animals. Let's say that this is an approach that not everyone can afford and that certainly could not guarantee adequate consumption for the growing world population. Of course we do not talk about bacon, cold meats or preserved meat. Consumption should be about fresh meat, with frequent use of offal such as liver, heart and bone marrow. Eggs are obviously included, in quantities that certainly would make those doctors who forbid them because of cholesterol fall out: we speak 6-12 eggs a week, strictly from hens raised outdoors.

Fish
Along with the meat on the tables of the devout Paleo should not miss good fish, strictly wild, preferably cold or blue water. Alaskan salmon is the holy Grail but the list includes virtually all

fish, crustaceans and molluscs you can get your hands on. Obviously these are foods with an excellent nutritional profile, source as well as excellent proteins also of good quality fats.

vegetable

From the leafy vegetables to the common vegetables all the vegetables are well received on the paleotavola, abundant, raw or cooked, as long as they are in season and possibly at zero kilometers, or so.

Fruit

Even for fruit there are no particular restrictions; with vegetables it is the main source of sugars in the diet.

Oil seeds and nuts

Nuts, hazelnuts, almonds, brazil nuts, pecans, pumpkin seeds and oil seeds are generally considered excellent sources of protein and are rich in the right fatty acids. Obviously, moderate use is recommended, given the rich caloric intake.

Oils and fats

Among the recommended oils, the olive oil - which is so paleo is not - and that of coconut, between the fatty lard and butter: obviously in controlled quantities and not dry, as recommended in some adventurous interpretations of the Paleolithic diet.

In most cases there is no mention of percentages related to the various nutrients: the experience suggests that the income of meat and fish can range from 20 to 40-60% in different populations. Surely most of the dish should be planted, with a good supply of fruit and fat. Very different from the coals of grilled bison lined with bacon that often pretend to paleo while they are simple attempts to suicide overweight Americans.

In the end the idea is to have a good supply of high quality proteins, around 1.2-1.5 grams per kg of body weight against 0.8 g / kg weight of the guidelines, a good supply of carbohydrates - from 25 to 50% - coming mainly from fruit and vegetables, and from a fat intake between 30 and 40%, with a ratio between omega6 and omega 3 moved towards the latter.

The foods to avoid are those that have appeared on our table with the passage to agriculture, foods consumed in a very occasional manner in the Paleolithic, domesticated and become the cornerstones of the Neolithic diet.

Cereals
Practically the source of all evil, the cereals must be eliminated in full: too rich in sugar, their consumption causes dramatic fluctuations in blood sugar, creates hormonal storms, sets the conditions for the accumulation of fat and the development is a pro-inflammatory state . In addition, cereals are rich in antinutrients such as phytates that inhibit the absorption of fats and vitamins, and obviously, at least some, contain gluten that can trigger severe immune problems.
Also included in the heap pseudo-cereal as amaranth, quinoa and buckwheat, also guilty, despite the significant and valuable protein intake, to be excessively rich in sugar.
legumes
The legumes would have the same dramatic effects of cereals, with an even greater antinutrient load: how to forget the lectins, certain oligosaccarians and some protease inhibitors. For the more fervent paleosostenitori consume a plate of beans is more or less equivalent to a death sentence, ultimately.
Tubers
The situation here is more nuanced: Cordain condemns them without appeal, like bombs of sugar waiting to explode in the jars of the unfortunate consumer, while Lindeberg, strong of his studies on Kitavani, very large consumers of tubers, with an iron health, admits consumption. Maybe you should avoid potatoes, preferring more exotic products from sweet potato, to tapioca, to taro.
Obviously, in the original formulation, all types of preserved meat - including bacon, a blow to the paleo-enthusiasts of America - meat, industrial products of all kinds, sweets, with the

exception of modest quantities, must be avoided like the plague. of honey, excess salt, vegetable oils and margarines.

Some of the closest observers also propose the elimination of some vegetables such as tomatoes and aubergines, rich in solanine, toxic substances that however are reduced with aging and are eliminated by cooking. There are many tribes and many food taboos, with some concession to taste and palate related to "comfort" kinds such as tea, coffee, chocolate - strictly melting - that are allowed in small quantities, as well as wine and spirits, which for some can be consumed, albeit with great measure.

The theses on which the paleo diet is based are undoubtedly suggestive, but not very solid and based on little precise and often debatable assumptions. In the first place, all the affirmations concerning the diet of our ancestors are difficult to verify, they are at best well circumstantiated hypotheses, while the few surviving hunter-gatherer tribes present food regimes very different from one another and strictly dependent on the nature of the territory.

As for cereals, some findings show that the cultivation and consumption of wheat are not as recent as hypothesized but could date back to over 100,000 years ago, with the use of flour of various types already widespread in Europe over 30,000 years ago . Legumes have also been part of the human diet for much longer than it was supposed to be.
Many studies show a positive contribution of cereals, whole species and legumes to a good state of health. On the other hand, the deficiencies due to phytates and other antinutrients present are rare, which can become significant only in very limited diets with reduced consumption or complete absence of food of animal origin. And it makes little sense to say that consumption of cereals and legumes by itself causes

inflammation and therefore is at the root of all evil. Inflammation in general is a symptom not a disease, and numerous studies have shown that while exaggerated consumption of refined grains may contribute to a systemic inflammation state adequate consumption of whole grains seems to have protective effect.

It should be noted that the much feared and demonized gluten causes real problems, and well diagnosed, to a very small percentage of the population, probably less than 1%, while it is still unclear whether or not gluten hypersensitivity exists which in any case would affect at most 10%. And it seems useless to point out that there are cereals and pseudo-cereals that are completely devoid of gluten, from rice to quinoa.

Regarding lectins and saponins, the fearsome poisons of legumes, which in the opinion of detractors would reduce to a sieve the wall of the intestine, causing the leaky gut syndrome, these are statements that have not been investigated at the moment with adequate studies , and it is therefore difficult to support correctness.

The other great accused in the paleo-supporter's court is milk, with all its derivatives. Let's start from the basic observation, the classic "only man consumes adult milk, and moreover of other species": evidently these gentlemen have never seen dogs or cats in the presence of milk and especially, in nature, different species work to recover milk from other animals.
Equally unfounded are the claims that milk is an "acidifier", milk and dairy products do not in fact produce acidic or metabolic acidosis, or cause osteoporosis, as proven by a large number of controlled studies. Among other things, the fact that a large part of the Western population, from 50 to 95% in Europe and North America, retains the activity of lactase, an enzyme essential for the digestion of milk even in adulthood rather than losing it in

childhood, as is still the case for most of the African and Asian populations, it is a very clear proof of how evolution and selection operate extremely rapidly in the human population, much faster than supposed by the paleo diet theorists who would like our genome frozen in some point of the remote past, 100 or 200,000 years ago. The domestication of dairy animals and the use of milk and its derivatives have given such an obvious advantage in the populations in which they occurred, to determine an effective selection of those individuals who retained the ability to digest these foods as adults. Individuals who then transmitted this character to their numerous offspring, determining a notable diffusion of these traits in the human population, relevant among those peoples for whom the consumption of milk was essential for survival in decidedly hostile environments: ask the Scandinavian friends.

For what concerns the fatty acids, certainly the research shows the importance of a good consumption of omega 3, but there are no specific relationships or doses. Indeed, many of the warmly recommended foods in the Paleo diet, such as coconut oil or almonds, have an omega 6 content - so dangerous for Paleo theorists - dramatically elevated compared to omega 3. Even here consumption is more important careful and varied, rather than a strenuous search for values that are little more than hypotheses.

And finally no, gentlemen, sugar is not a deadly white poison, refined and lethal ready to disintegrate the wall of your vessels. As always is the dose that makes the poison and if you like a teaspoon of refined sugar in the coffee, which of course is not paleo since there were no espresso machines in the savannah during the Paleolithic, use it. If you consume industrial quantities of desserts, make an examination of conscience, but not because you eat non-pale foods: simply because you eat too much and badly.

These observations have the sole purpose of highlighting how some "theoretical" bases of the paleo diet are not correct and derive from unproven assumptions or even in contrast with the available data. This does not deny that some assumptions are interesting and that indeed the modern Western diet is unsuitable for our lifestyle, but more for reasons related to excess and poor quality of food than to the specific type of food consumed. Certainly we are not well adapted to our current lifestyle, as the biologist Daniel Lieberman writes in his The History of the Human Body, but the situation is much more nuanced and complex than painted with rather imprecise brushes by the proponents of the paleo diet.

And I do not want to talk about the grotesque market of paleo supplements based on milk proteins or maltodextrin that should perhaps replace fresh but very forbidding foods, a veritable fair of bad faith. Always be wary of diets that require you to permanently renounce whole food groups, tracing a clear line between good and bad foods. Man is an omnivorous and much of his evolutionary success is due precisely to his ability to adapt to diets and deeply different foods. Except the hemlock, which hurts even if it is natural.

Maybe reading the article gives the impression of a certain skepticism on my part towards this approach to food but it is not so. Personally I am fascinated by the paleo diet and the theoretical bases on which it rests, however I am annoyed by the dogmatisms and assumptions passed off for scientific certainties.

The theoretical approach of the paleo diet is to identify, in the sphere of nutrition, those foods that in the light of our history are the most suitable for our genetic heritage, discarding those that could instead be a problem. Excellent concept on paper whose application in the field is much more difficult and complex, as we have seen. However, after an initial period of skepticism, mainly due to the excesses of overly enthusiastic supporters, the academic world has begun to examine the Palaeolithic diet, investigating its possible applications in those areas that appear to be most promising, especially Diabetes type 2 and cardiovascular diseases.

The results of various interventions on sedentary and overweight subjects showed, even in very short periods, a marked improvement in parameters related to metabolic well-being and cardiovascular risk, with a reduction in the various indices linked to the metabolic syndrome, in particular pressure and hyperlipidemia. It is interesting that in some interventions in which paleo diet and a balanced diet were compared, both designed to maintain the weight of the subjects constant, in individuals who were feeding paleo it was recorded however a significant weight loss.

The results of studies conducted on subjects with type 2 diabetes were very interesting: the paleo diet showed a better glycemic control and a greater sensation of satiety, an improvement of the lipid profile and insulin sensitivity with a greater weight loss and a more marked improvement of several important metabolic indices compared to a traditional diabetic diet. Results that could, in selected subjects and with well-studied food plans, suggest a possible use of this diet in the treatment of diabetes.

There are no studies related to other diseases for which the enthusiastic proponents of the paleo see applications harbingers of amazing results: there are no jobs that affect the effect of a paleolithic diet in individuals with cancer or in patients with autoimmune diseases. Protocols for the treatment of tumors or diseases such as Multiple Sclerosis with paleo-inspired diets circulate in the network: these are protocols that have no scientific validation and for which no studies have been carried out. It is therefore good to be wary of it, at least until we have available real and measurable data and not anecdotal reports without any scientific value.

Just as we must not particularly trust the enthusiastic accounts of subjects who, thanks to the paleo, have obtained miraculous results: they are often individuals whose lifestyle and diet was so compromised that the simple introduction of good quantities of vegetables and fruit and the overall reduction of the caloric intake associated with a well-behaved paleo can significantly improve the initial conditions.

However, one should not even demonize the paleo as the diet of carnivores, confusing picturesque as demeaning degenerations with the protocol initially suggested for example by Lindeberg and Cordain. In the end it is a diet in which the bulk of the food intake is represented by fruits and vegetables, including tubers, with important shares of meat and fish and quality fats, from olive oil to seeds and nuts. One could, and generally does, much worse. My inner neanderthal is happy.

Chapter 2: Eat food, not nutrients

Bread and pasta? They contain gluten. Meat? Only proteins. Fruit? Oh my God, the sugars! However, red wine is good because it contains resveratrol. And the wheat germ? so rich in precious fats. And the chocolate then, is full of antioxidants! When we stop talking about food and we focus only on nutrients we lose sight of what really matters in nutrition, ending up considering every food as the simple sum of the substances that compose it, an error that leads to eating in an unbalanced way , often bordering on orthorexia.

It often happens to read or hear experts and nutrition gurus who recommend eating a food because it is rich in betaine or quercetin, while certain foods should be avoided because they can contain aflatoxins, mercury, phytates and other anti-nutrients. And based on the content of this or that component, on the presence or absence of a certain nutrient or a substance considered dangerous, more or less restrictive diets arise, in which certain foods are favored at the expense of others, trying to optimize the 'taking this or that compound miraculous properties, hoping to minimize the consumption of those substances that are considered dangerous.

Those who follow this kind of indications end up considering food as simply a collection of substances each of which has a positive or negative effect, the effect on which one chooses to consume it or not. An approach that reduces every food to the sum of its components, exposing those who follow it to risks and errors that are probably worse than the problems you are trying to avoid.

Someone has read somewhere that legumes contain phytates. And that the terrible, terrible phytates can interfere with the absorption of iron and other minerals. And then completely eliminates all the legumes from their diet, neglecting the fact that not only a normal consumption of legumes does not create particular problems with regard to the intake of iron but can have positive effects on numerous risk factors for cardiovascular diseases, with reduction of inflammation markers and a decisive antioxidant action that is partly due to the action of the feared phytates, which also have a protective action against some cancers.

Avoiding legumes and other vegetables that contain them for fear of phytates is nonsense, just as it is to remove all the cereals that contain gluten when there is no real need, so, just to follow the latest food fad. Of course, it is easy to suggest that all the problems a person complains about are attributable to a single, tremendous enemy: a simple and suggestive solution that allows you to download any responsibility today on the fitati, tomorrow on gluten, then on palm oil and so on, from enemy to enemy, but without trying to intervene in a clear and decisive manner on one's lifestyle.

And this way of reasoning is also perfect to generate a huge market of targeted products and diets that isolate specific nutrients or substances, responsible for all wickedness and to be avoided anyway. The risk is that those who follow these imaginative directions find themselves believing that in the end it is safe and protected from all evil and that having eliminated the "bad nutrient" can afford everything, because nothing can create problems: situation that often occurs between the followers of the food without, those who choose to remove because so they take shelter from the evils caused by the enemy on duty.

Bruce Ames, a leading scholar to whom we owe one of the most used tests to determine whether or not a substance can be considered carcinogenic, goes so far as to argue that concern about the presence of pesticides in the vegetables and fruit we consume - widespread concern today - is a false problem and may even be harmful because it could lead to limiting the consumption of these foods, essential for our health, due to an absolutely modest risk but perceived, unfortunately, as enormous.

The diametrically opposite position is that of those who consider certain nutrients or substances present in some food as the perfect cure for every illness. From time to time it is lemon, ginger and turmeric to solve even the most thorny health situations, real miracle foods.

Often the indications regarding the use of these nutrients are derived from studies on cell cultures or work on animals, the lowest degree of scientific evidence, passed instead for final and astonishing results instead of preliminary data, simple bases on which to build new and more accurate research phases, which are instead.

In this way, the promotion of the rich food of the "miraculous nutrient" takes place, a real elixir of long life, to be consumed anyway. This is good, otherwise it triggers the promotion of supplements as expensive as little or not at all useful, in which the substance is concentrated in industrial quantities, in the wrong belief, so dear to American friends, if ten is good then center it will do better, much better. Dangerous conviction, because many of the substances promoted in this sense can have very problematic effects if taken in too high quantities, able to interfere with specific processes of our organism. Or, simply, you can bring many, too many calories: it is the case of dark chocolate or extra virgin olive oil, real nutrient mines whose positive action is proven beyond doubt but that if consumed in large quantities can have a major impact on the overall caloric balance.

A classic case are certain antioxidants even promoted as the cure against aging thanks to their action of contrasting the fearful free radicals, a very gross simplification of a reality that is much more complex and dynamic, based on the subtle balance between antioxidants and reactive species that, far from being just a problem, have very precise and really important roles in our body. Entering the stretched leg in these dynamics, without having carefully assessed their real needs, is not exactly a good idea, as evidenced by the fact that supplementation with antioxidants can even have negative effects on athletic performance.

When the search for certain "positive" nutrients pushes us to change our diet, when the attention to certain problematic substances induces us to reflect on our eating habits without necessarily distorting them, then more information on what is present in our dishes can become a real positive factor, able to improve our lifestyle.

If instead we discard a priori certain foods because they contain nutrients or dangerous substances, if we are to consume almost exclusively some foods because they are rich in this or that miraculous nutrient, then the situation is getting out of hand and our crusade for a food healthy is becoming a real problem, a somewhat less severe form of orthorexia.

My suggestion and my conviction are that rather than dealing with single nutrients, rather than measuring every single substance we consume in an obsessive way, we pay attention first of all to the overall balance of our diet and lifestyle. The real, important and real risks are smoking, alcohol, overweight and sedentary: once we are aware of this and that we intervene where the enormous, real and important problems are really, we could try to optimize other aspects of our diet that in our head appear to be decisive but often have a marginal or even negligible impact.

A diet based on vegetables, with a fair supply of whole grains and legumes, quality meat and fish, dairy products, olive oil and dried fruit is important, but it is even more important that this nutrition is measured and never excessive, that our body weight is normal, that there is a good dose of physical activity every day, that you avoid smoking and that the consumption of alcohol is absolutely occasional. Here is the bulk of the work to be done. Breaking the attention from the heart of the problem to minor details, creating unjustified alarms and hopes, certainly does not serve our health, but certainly makes those who fear and speculate on us happy.

We try to consider what we eat for what it is, not as a simple sum of nutrients, with an emotional and cultural value, without exhausting all our anxieties and obsessions, our faults and our hopes. We will eat better and, probably, we will live better.

Chapter 3: The quality of your proteins

Amino acids are the building blocks of proteins, large molecules whose structure and functions are due precisely to the sequence of the amino acids that compose them. Proteins are nutrients of great importance for our body but not all proteins are the same: some have more value than others, a higher biological value that makes them precious.

Amino acids are carbon compounds characterized, unlike fats and sugars, by the presence of nitrogen atoms in their molecule. The structure is simple: a central carbon atom binds an amino group -NH2, a carboxylic group -COOH, a hydrogen atom and a side chain - denoted by the letter R - which is different in each of the known amino acids. It is estimated that there are about 500 amino acids in nature but only 20 of these are present in proteins and are coded by triplets of bases - called codons - at the DNA level.

The amino group imparts basic properties to the molecule, while the carboxylic acid determines acidic properties, whereby the amino acids are amphoteric molecules, which have both acid and basic behavior: at physiological pH - between 7.3 and 7.4 - both groups they are ionized, that is, equipped with charge. Amino acids are bound together by a peptide bond that is formed between the carboxyl group of an amino acid and the amino group of a second amino acid, a condensation reaction that can be repeated several times leading to the formation of long chains of amino acids that when they exceed 20-30 units are called proteins.

The sequence of amino acids determines the way in which protein chains fold and organize themselves in space, their shape on which their specific function depends.

Amino acids can be classified in many different ways, depending on the characteristics that are taken into consideration. If we consider them from the biochemical point of view, it is extremely useful to classify them according to the polarity of the side chain, a classification that allows us to understand the role that the single amino acids have in determining the three-dimensional structure of the protein they are part of:

Amino acids with apolar neutral lateral chain: alanine, phenylalanine, glycine, isoleucine, leucine, methionine, proline, tyrosine, tryptophan, valine;
Amino acids with a polar neutral lateral chain: asparagine, glutamine, serine, threonine, cysteine;
Amino acids with side chain, acidic charge: aspartate (aspartic acid), glutamate (glutamic acid);
Amino acids with a basic charge side chain: arginine, histidine, lysine.
For those interested in nutrition, the classification based on the fate of the amino acids present in foods is much more useful. The proteins in the food consumed are in fact digested and decomposed into the amino acids that constitute them, amino acids that are then absorbed and that can be used at the cellular level both for synthesis processes and for metabolic processes.

From the metabolic point of view amino acids can be distinguished in:

ketogenic aminoacids, which as a final product of their metabolism give a molecule of acetylCoA, which can be used to produce ketone bodies: leucine, lysine;

glucogenic amino acids, which as a final product of their metabolism give substances that can be used for:

produce glucose: alanine, cysteine, glycine, serine and threonine;

substances that can be used in place of glucose in the energy processes of the cell: arginine, aspartic acid, glutamic acid, asparagine, glutamine, histidine, methionine, proline, tyrosine, valine;

mixed amino acids, which can give both glucose and acetylCoA precursors: isoleucine, phenylalanine, threonine, tryptophan and serine.

Amino acids can therefore participate in the regulation of cellular energy processes and can be used to produce energy instead of glucose or fatty acids in particular situations, especially when the availability of glucose is reduced.

The best known classification of amino acids is based on the body's ability to synthesize a given molecule or not.

The essential amino acids are those that we must necessarily take with the diet, since we are not able to synthesize them starting from precursors or because the existing synthetic pathways are not able to meet the needs that the organism presents for that substance.

There are non-essential amino acids that we can instead produce in an autonomous way and in an adequate quantity for the needs of the organism.

Essentially essential amino acids are those that can only become essential in some particular situations, for example in premature individuals, during childhood or in conditions of strong catabolic stress.

Some amino acids can be converted into each other and are defined as semi-essential because the body can still synthesize them from other essential amino acids if present in quantities greater than the requirement: the phenylalanine can be converted into tyrosine in the liver, while methionine can be used to produce cysteine.

The availability of amino acids is a limiting factor for protein synthesis processes that can be blocked due to the lack of a single essential amino acid. In the sports field are used many integrations with the three branched amino acids, leucine, isoleucine and valine, with the leucine that plays a key role as a messenger able to activate the transcription of specific genes involved in protein synthesis processes and to participate in processes of regulation of the mechanisms involved in the synthesis of proteins.

Even for essential amino acids there are recommended daily intake levels and over the past 20 years the World Health Organization has repeatedly reviewed and modified these values.

We have seen that not all amino acids are the same: some, the essentials, for our body are definitely more precious than others. Some works even seem to indicate that a good consumption of essential amino acids can be considered a protective factor while an excessive consumption of non-essential amino acids could even have a negative effect: a very interesting field of study that could present really interesting developments

In order to objectively evaluate the quality or value of different types of proteins, several methods have been proposed:

Biological value of proteins

Measure the amount of protein in the consumed food that is absorbed and incorporated into the proteins of the person who consumes that food. It is a complex indicator to measure but very practical and widely used in different fields. However it has limits, it is in fact strongly dependent on the amino acid composition of the protein and above all the lack of essential amino acids that are obviously limiting factors for protein synthesis processes. It is also influenced by the cooking method and the presence of vitamins and minerals that can alter the availability and absorption of the amino acids present. In general it is indicated with respect to a reference food, the egg, which contains proteins that are considered to be immediately used by the body.

Protein digestibility
Measure how much a certain protein is digested, is given by the ratio between absorbed and ingested nitrogen

Protein efficiency ratio
Indicates the weight gain for each gram of protein ingested, in subjects maintained in standardized nutritional conditions.

Net protein use
It is given by the ratio between the amino acids converted into proteins and those consumed with the diet, a measure of the amount of ingested nitrogen that is retained by the body.

Appropriate protein digestibility score from limiting amino acid (PDCAAS)
Introduced by the World Health Organization in 1993, it is based on the comparison of the amino acid profile of the test protein with a reference amino acid profile: the maximum score is 1 and indicates that the studied protein provides 100% of the required amount of the essential amino acid considered. This value takes into account the real human needs for each essential amino acid

and the digestibility of the protein, with some limitations due to differences in absorption and the presence of anti-nutritional factors that may partially alter the values obtained.

Score of the digestibility of essential amino acids (DIAAS)
Proposed by the World Health Organization in 2013 to replace PDCAAS, takes into account the digestion and absorption of amino acids in the protein in the small intestine, is therefore more accurate and less error prone than the other methods.

Each of these methods has advantages and defects. On the whole they allow to evaluate with good approximation the goodness of the proteins present in different foods and above all, when the values are not particularly high - as happens for proteins of vegetable origin that often have a reduced content of some essential amino acids - make it possible to suggest combinations that they make up for the specific shortcomings of the individual foods. Some combinations that give a PDCAAS equal to 1, starting from foods that have reduced values, are:

Rice and peas
Cereals and legumes
Cereals and vegetables
Cereals, nuts and seeds
Legumes, nuts and seeds
Rice and milk

It is not difficult to recognize among these combinations popular dishes of our tradition: rice and pasta and beans, for example, choices that next to the taste andavasno to meet the physiological needs of our body, making a virtue of necessity. Let's remember it when it comes to the biological value of proteins, without constantly referring to meat or milk proteins, which are simply some of the many possible choices, not always the best ones.

Chapter 4: Is meat really that bad?

For a vegan the link between cancer and meat is a fact. For the adept of the paleo diet, meat, as long as it is grazed, is the healthiest food in the world and the risk is also linked to exaggerated consumption. In the middle there are so many problems that arise, but they are often confused by exaggerated titles and studies with mixed results.

The consumption of meat in the world is constantly increasing, even if there are significant differences between the western countries, where it reaches an average consumption of 23kg per person per year, and those in development, where it stops at just 6kg a head by year. Studies on different populations, or migrant ethnic groups, have shown a significant difference in the incidence of different types of cancer and different lifestyles.

Hundreds of epidemiological studies have investigated the possible link between certain types of cancer and nutrition. These studies are difficult to perform due to the difficulty of collecting data, usually through questionnaires on the consumption of certain foods, subject to possible errors and inaccuracies of the participants, both due to the influence that many other factors of lifestyle of the subjects studied on the topic: for example, strong consumers of red meat and preserved are also strong fat consumers, often overweight, with poor diets of fruit and vegetables. In these subjects, in the face of a higher incidence of some types of cancer, it is difficult to disentangle between the effect of each of the different behaviors at risk.

When we talk about cancer we must also consider that we are talking about a complex disease with a common root: mutations that allow cells to replicate freely and quickly. Mutations that become more and more frequent as the body ages with much greater incidence in the elderly population, so much so that some researchers believe that at least one third of the tumors can arise due to "bad luck", as Vogelstein and Tomasetti say in a very criticized article. Certainly the incidence of some types of cancer is certainly linked to certain behaviors, lung cancer and cigarette smoking for example, but for other cancers the link with specific lifestyles is a subject of strong discussion and careful investigation. The current consensus is that at least 40/50% of tumors can be attributed to lifestyles and modifiable environmental factors: of course, there are no diets or behaviors that can completely eliminate the risk of getting sick, but given the influence that our choices they may have, it is worth paying attention.

The meat is generally divided into three different types:

fresh red dog: meat from cattle, sheep and pigs that have not been processed. This category generally also includes game and game meat. These are meat with a high iron content;
processed meat: all types of meat that have undergone some kind of processing from ham, sausages, frankfurters, bacon and industrial meat products. In general, additives of a different nature are used, often nitrites;
white meat: chicken, turkey and rabbit meat, generally characterized by a reduced iron content.
Not all studies take into account the differences listed above, especially the older ones. However, it has been found that it is very important to collect data carefully evaluating the type of meat that we want to assess the impact on cancer risk and many specific studies exist on the topic.

Archaeological finds show that cancer is a very old disease, as evidenced by the numerous findings of old bone tens of thousands of years with obvious cancerous lesions. Of course we do not know much about soft tissue tumors and very little of the risk factors present in the environment of these ancestral populations; we can hypothesize that the absolute incidence of tumors was inferior to the current one, above all due to the high mortality in young age.

Rural populations show a lower incidence than western ones, with the risk for specific types of cancer, colon, lung, breast, prostate, which varies appreciably between different cultures; a fact that reinforces the hypothesis that the risk of contracting these diseases is linked to diet and lifestyle.

There are hundreds of epidemiological and observational studies on the subject and numerous reviews and meta-analyzes that attempted to summarize the results of these studies.

Tumors of the colon and rectum
According to numerous works there seems to be a link between high consumption of red and processed meat and colorectal tumors, with an effect that seems to depend on the dose: the risk is increasing, the extent of the increase in incidence is estimated in fact around 28% for every 100g of meat consumed, 9% for every 30g. Not all studies give clear data, the link with colon cancer seems stronger, while the one with rectal cancer seems to be less or weak. The consumption of white meat does not seem to have any connection with this type of cancer.

Stomach and pancreas tumors
Once again a growing consumption of red and processed dog seems to increase the incidence of tumors of the stomach and pancreas. Some studies show that consumption of more than 100g per day of red meat triples the risk of stomach cancer. The increase recorded for pancreatic tumors, around 40%, especially for processed meats, is also important.

Lung cancer
The number of studies on the topic is less, but a recent meta-analysis has shown that there is an association between

consumption of red meat and increased incidence of lung cancer. The association is very attenuated in subjects that consume in quantity fruit and vegetables, and it seems to be weaker for the meat worked. White meat shows a very weak protective effect.

Prostate cancer
In this case the association is weak, higher for processed meat, almost negligible for fresh red meat. No correlation for white meat.

Breast cancer
The observed association is very weak, statistically not significant. Existing sutds show disparities depending on the status of estrogen and progesterone receptors and indicate the need for further investigation.

The situation for other types of tumors, such as the liver, is less nuanced, less investigated in this respect. Interesting are the two studies below that investigate the situation for various types of cancer in the world and in America.

Studies show that consumption of red meat and processed meat can present a quantifiable risk for various cancers. Several possible hypothetical mechanisms of action:

red meat contains a high amount of iron in heme form. It is an iron with strong pro-oxidative activity, able to cause strong lipid peroxidation and to cause DNA damage in different tissues. This mechanism is particularly important for lung and colorectal cancers. The degradation of nitrogen compounds by specific bacterial strains in the colon can lead to the formation of ammonia and other nitrogen-containing compounds (NOCs), strong promoters of carcinogenesis. The addition of nitrites, common in the preparation of preserved meat, can encourage their formation. This effect can be further increased by the presence of heme iron and decreased significantly in the presence of a high fiber content. Cooking at high temperatures of the meat, on the grill or on the grill, leads to the formation of heterocyclic amines (HCA). These compounds are formed by the reaction between creatine, amino acids and sugars and show a significant activity of carcinogenesis in the intestine and to a lesser extent of the prostate and the breast. The heterocyclic amines to bind to the DNA and start the carcinogenesis must be activated by the enzyme N-acetyltransferase (NAT) that in different subjects has different speeds, with greater risk for those with high-speed enzymes. The presence of this different answer could explain the discrepancy of the results in different studies.

cooking at elevated temperatures, especially when extended areas are burnt or charred, can also lead to the formation of polycyclic aromatic hydrocarbons that once absorbed into the cell can bind to DNA forming adducts that promote carcinogenesis and interfere with apoptosis, cell death, important mechanism that prevents the uncontrolled proliferation of cells.

some types of red and processed meat may have a high fat content which leads to an increase in bile salts released into the intestinal lumen and to an increase in their degradation product by the bacterial flora of the colon, the deoxycholic acid; this compound stimulates the proliferation of the colon mucosa and can act as a promoter of the development of cancer cells. The possible association between the fat content of the diet and the increase in the incidence of certain types of tumors remains controversial.

a possible mechanism could be linked to the increase of IGF-1, an insulin-bound hormone, determined by the consumption of diets rich in animal proteins and a strong promoter of cell division processes. Studies in this regard have yielded controversial results with a modest increase in risk for prostate cancers and breast cancers in pre-menopausal women. Some particular monosaccharides, the sialic acids, are absent in our cells but present in the cells of many of the mammals used for meat production. Some of these acids, such as Neu5Gc, can cause an inflammatory response in our body, a process that could play some role in the development of cancer cells. This is a hypothesis that has just been outlined, which requires more detailed studies to be confirmed.

Let's start from a fact: vegetarians and vegans have a modest reduction in the risk of contracting certain types of cancer, about 18%, even if some meta-analyzes have not shown appreciable differences. Some have even pointed out that the maximum risk reduction is not between vegetarians and vegans but between subjects that essentially consume fish. To renounce completely to meat does not therefore seem to confer decisive protection against these diseases.

The relationship between red meat, processed meat and cancer exists, but there are many factors that can determine it: fat content, type and extent of cooking processes, simultaneous consumption of vegetables, more or less healthy lifestyle. In general it would be advisable to consume fresh, lean red meat, in quantities not exceeding 100g daily, no more than 3 or 4 times a week, avoiding cooking at high temperatures that can burn or burn the meat.
Consumption of processed meat, from sausages to various industrial products, should be reduced in quantity and above all in terms of frequency, limiting it to quality products and special occasions.

White meat does not seem to represent a particular risk factor, indeed in some studies they showed a weak protective effect. Even here, however, it is appropriate to choose lean cuts and avoid cooking that can burn or carbonize the meat leading to the development of potentially carcinogenic compounds.

Who eats meat should avoid other potential risk factors, such as smoking and alcohol, and should try to consume a good amount and variety of vegetables and fruit, which have shown an important protective action against these diseases, maintaining a normal body weight and practicing adequate physical activity.

Meat has always been a sought-after and precious food for all human cultures. I do not think we should give it up. However, a more responsible consumption is necessary both for environmental reasons and for our personal health: eating meat choosing quality rather than quantity, paying attention to how it is cooked and stored, is one of the strategies that can protect us from those diseases that have become now sinister companions of well-being and abundance.

Chapter 5: Paleo Diet vs Detox Diet

You can call them whatever you want, purifying diets, detoxifying diets, detoxifying diets, detox if you are really trendy. The idea is that your body has become saturated with unspecified toxins, dirt, tired, covered with mucus and other horrors, and that it takes a long period of penance to give a good cleaning to all: especially after the holidays . But do these exercises in deprivation and renunciation really serve something?

Every new year opens under the banner of the most imaginative detox diets. The sense of guilt for the excesses related to the holidays is strong and you try to run for cover, choosing among the myriad of proposed protocols, hoping to cancel the damage done, removing in the quickest way all the horrible toxins accumulated in fifteen days of follies. The common trait of detoxifying diets is absolute rigidity, a brutal restriction that in extreme cases is based on juices, a handful of fruit and vegetables and little else. Lemon and ginger are never lacking, perhaps accompanied by cayenne pepper (you do not want to use regular pepper?), A little minestrone, vegetables, extracts, legumes and herbal teas, liters of herbal teas. Beware of fruit that is saturated with frightful fructose, never foods of animal origin - if you insist, a filet of pitched steam - and, ça va sans dire, strictly gluten-free cereals.

Those who propose these diets say that by following these draconian measures our body will get rid of any accumulated toxin, will lose weight without any problem and, while we are there, will return healthy and beautiful, erasing every ailment and illness. Wonderful! And there are famous celebrities to be celebrated that will decant the benefits they have had from this or that detox diet. Too bad that moving from the golden world of the rich and famous to that a little less glamorous, but certainly more attentive to data, scientific research are lacking solid elements to support these depurative baldness.

For the proponents of detoxification, the term includes any substance that is believed to create problems in our body, with particular attention to synthetic products - the dreaded chemicals. Chemical additives, dyes, contaminants such as heavy metals and pesticides, preservatives, sweeteners, are constantly in the dock, alongside natural products of metabolism, free radicals, urea, mucus, pus and so on: this is the progressive accumulation of these substances to create problems and only an adequate detox diet can eliminate them before they do damage.

Undoubtedly many of the substances that appear on the lists of professional detoxifiers are actually problematic: it must always be clarified in which quantity and with which frequency of consumption. The context is important.

In many cases the tests of the dangerousness of a substance come from in vitro studies or on an animal model, with very high concentrations of the compound under examination, values that can not be achieved in real life. It must be kept in mind that in sufficiently high quantities, even water can be a problem for our body and can cause acute and potentially lethal intoxication. Even those fantastic mineral salts that are almost obligatory in summer, to get a little higher, have their dark side: a high potassium intake, in particular conditions, can cause hyperkalemia, a situation characterized by cardiac arrhythmias, even mortal. In addition, toxic substances for some animal species are not for humans: did you know that the theobromine present in chocolate is potentially deadly for dogs? And that conjugated linoleic acid, a mixture of fatty acids that according to some studies could help lose weight, in rats causes serious liver problems?

There are many substances that have been identified as a potential cause of problems. For many of these, maximum tolerability limits have been established that can be taken on a daily basis without creating problems, and these are generally values that, if they are incorrect, are due to excess of caution. It is the case of pesticides and other contaminants, whose presence in food is constantly monitored (I have talked here and here).

Depending on their chemical nature certain substances can actually accumulate in certain tissues, causing problems in the long run. This is the case of heavy metals such as mercury, lead, arsenic, cadmium, chromium. These are real dangers which, however, are not to be magnified beyond measure. Because of the fear of mercury, there are subjects that completely eliminate fish from their diet, depriving themselves of precious nutrients for fear of a very remote risk (an article with some more details on fish and mercury).

And as regards certain products of metabolic processes, it is clear that our body is perfectly capable of managing them or we would not be here to discuss these so suggestive themes.

To hear the supporters of detox would be believed that the human body is totally defenseless against the ongoing assault of toxic substances to which it is subjected. Not so: liver, kidneys, lungs, intestines and other organs work hard, every single moment, to remove toxic substances and metabolic waste.

Two classes of enzymes play an important role, those of phase I and those of phase II, whose role is crucial in detoxification processes.

Class I enzymes catalyze oxidation, reduction and hydrolysis reactions: an important role is played by the superfamily of cytochrome P450, a group of enzymes mainly present in the liver as well as in the intestine, lungs and brain, very active towards xenobiotics (a technical term that identifies any substance foreign to the body), steroid hormones and drugs.

The final product of the action of the enzymes of class I is a substance that can still present problems and which is inactivated thanks to the action of class II enzymes, enzymes whose function is to transfer hydrophilic groups - highly affinity for the water - on the product to be removed, which can then be excreted through the bile or urine. Enzymes of this group are glucuronosyltransferases, sulfotransferases, glutathione-S-transferases, N-acetyltransferases and methyltransferases.

The metallotienins, a group of proteins involved in the metabolism of some essential minerals such as zinc and copper, play a very important role. These proteins, found mainly in the liver and kidneys, can bind heavy metals and also participate in the neutralization of free radicals and the reduction of oxidative stress.

Many of these enzymes are inducible: their presence in the cell can increase or decrease in response to the consumption of specific foods. Phytonutrients such as sulforafano present in cruciferous, resveratrol, curcumin, some substances in tea, quercetin, the many bioactive substances of garlic and onion, can increase or decrease the activity of the enzymes of the cytochrome P450 family and a similar effect it is observed, with these and other substances, also on class II enzymes.

The expression of class II enzymes is regulated by a transcription factor, Nrf2, whose activity can be modulated by the phytonutrients of tea, coffee, turmeric, ginger, soy, pomegranate, citrus and broccoli; several studies have shown a greater effectiveness of the protective action of detoxification enzymes in correspondence with a high consumption of certain foods rich in these phytonutrients.

For detoxification enzymes there is a high polymorphism, there are different forms of the genes that code for these proteins and therefore different forms of each enzyme, each with different activity.

The picture is therefore very complex, with an effective defense against most of the toxic substances with which we come into contact. Defense that presents a remarkable genetic variability, on which we can not affect in any way (at least in the current state of knowledge); the effectiveness of defense can be modulated through diet, not through fasts and privations, but by consuming foods rich in those substances that can stimulate the activity of this battery of enzymes.

Finding that not everything is a toxin and that our body has its beautiful line of defense against substances that are really problematic, it remains to be determined whether the much-vaunted detox diets based on juices and vegetables really work.

If you look at scientific research, the answer is definitely negative. The studies are not very numerous and the few available often are on a too small number of subjects, with non-standardized protocols, usually in the absence of control groups and often based on qualitative and subjective measurements, rather than on quantitative data (ex. I feel better with the diet against measuring changes in a specific parameter, such as serum homocysteine).

The few randomized trials with control groups showed no appreciable differences between the effects recorded with a typical lemon and ginger detox diet and a normal diet with a similar caloric restriction.

Even in studies that have recorded the improvement of some specific parameters - fat mass, insulin resistance, C reactive protein - the authors point out that all the positive effects detected can be simply attributed to the caloric restriction typical of these diets, usually very rigid.

In practice, the trick is there and it is also in evidence: the benefits that are often enthusiastically reported by the subjects who undergo these fashionable diets are simply due to the severe reduction of caloric intake with an increase in consumption of fruit and vegetables . You lose weight quickly with these diets - beware: weight not fat! - and it increases the consumption of vitamins and micronutrients, present in plants, which may have been previously consumed in smaller quantities. Obviously it feels better, the diet seems to have worked: but there are risks.

Here we are talking about those diets that you find a lot to the kilo on the most diverse media, extreme diets made of deprivation, industrial quantities of water and lemon, some random spice and sparse meals based on juices and supplements, the detox Pop of the stars to be clear.

Scientific support is non-existent but potential problems are well documented: ranging from the most trivial ones such as weakness, migraine, strong fatigue, to the most severe, especially in subjects who may have some health problems, take drugs regularly, and have not considered the possible consequences of such rigid regimes.

Many of these diets propose the consumption in industrial quantities of supplements that contain a bit of everything - and generally have significant costs - often also diuretics and laxatives that could cause dehydration and alterations in the water-salt balance, or require the consumption of exotic food, rare spices, berries from the fabulous jungles of the East and Amazonia - at least some nice purifying herbal tea - and so on, in a riot of purchases as expensive as useless, which certainly purify only one thing: your bank account, from the money present.

With such rigid regimes, in which a good part of the commonly consumed foods is labeled as potentially dangerous, source of poisons and threats, we risk also to slip into problematic behaviors from the social point of view, up to arrive, in extreme cases, to real eating disorders, with creeping forms of orthorexia nervosa.

Fortunately, these are short cycles, because they are unsustainable over the long term; unfortunately, also the benefits observed are short and transient: the lost weight, water more than fat, is recovered quickly and moreover we have not worked to create healthy eating habits, indeed, in many cases the relationship with food has deteriorated further, moving from exaggerated consumption to waivers informed by fears and paranoia. A constant swing that makes it impossible to find any balance, an essential element of a healthy lifestyle.

The most pop detox diets are, more or less, the crafty commercial foundations, created to exploit our anxieties and our fears, our desire to achieve results in the shortest possible time, our feelings of guilt due to a problematic relationship with food and, more in general, with the stressful environment around us.

Better stay away.

If you really want to help your body - which is still doing well on its own - to manage the load of problematic substances coming from the environment more effectively, there are few simple but really useful things you can do.

keep well hydrated, remember to drink, water is essential for the proper functioning of our excretory organs, those that eliminate xenobiotics and by-products of the metabolism;
eat fresh food, rich in water and nutrients and not in calories;
keep a good consumption of green leafy vegetables, spinach, chard, cabbage and salads;
try to consume with a certain frequency garlic, onion, leeks and crucifers such as broccoli, cauliflower, savoy cabbage, brussels sprouts: they are rich in those compounds that stimulate the activity of the enzymes responsible for detoxification processes;
consume a fair amount of fruit. There are not only apples, pears, oranges and kiwis. And lemons. Instead, try to rotate fruit consumption by following the seasonality of the various products, perhaps with a special touch, occasionally: pomegranates, blueberries and berries, pineapples and so on. I would prefer the fruit, rather than the much-vaunted extracts: we avoid concentrating the sugars and throwing away some fibers that instead have a precious role in our diet;
use more spices, not necessarily cayenne pepper and ginger, and less salt. Excellent herbs of our tradition such as sage, thyme and rosemary, perhaps accompanied by a splash of the most exotic, from curry to cinnamon;
try to guarantee a good supply of vitamins and minerals, in particular calcium, iron, selenium, zinc and magnesium;
if you have to lose weight try to create a moderate caloric deficit, not by unnecessarily demonizing certain foods. Do not look for a forced loss of weight by completely eliminating the dreaded carbohydrates or hated fats: it does not work. Instead, try to eat in a balanced way with a good protein intake, quality

fats, especially olive oil and the amount of carbo necessary for your level of activity;

exercise regularly, keep yourself active. A sedentary lifestyle is a serious risk, as is being overweight.

I hope you do not think that fifteen days of penance can remedy the problems created by a wrong lifestyle. Rather than craving for a miraculous solution, try to have a healthy and balanced diet, adapted to your needs, be active and control the stress. Your organism thinks of the toxins effectively. Be wary of those who sell powders, extracts and concoctions, clays and coals, coffee enemas and various amenities, especially as the price is higher. If you think you have real problems, contact your doctor or a food professional, and do not mess around with these "purifying" toys, which can also be dangerous.

Then if you really want, that nice glass of lemon, ginger and pepper (of Cayenna, I recommend), drink it too: but do not expect miracles.

Chapter 6: Why you are not losing weight with the paleo diet

To lose weight it is not enough to cut the calories wildly and move more. Indeed, a strategy of this type can be counterproductive, due to the upheavals that cause the delicate hormonal balance of the organism, especially in cortisol.
A good part of the people who undertake a diet does not do it for health reasons: the goal is to recover the line, the physical form, often idealized, perhaps in reduced times and with maximum effectiveness. So often we witness a voluntary calorie restriction, we eat less, much less. It may also increase physical activity, in particular aerobic exercise, "cardio" for the more fashionable ones, spending hours and hours between treadmills, elittic, spinning lessons and other such amenities. And then, after the first exciting initial successes, the drama: weight loss stops, the general condition worsens and even the dreaded fat can go back up.

The picture described is well known by many women and is a source of great frustration and discouragement. Often in an attempt to overcome the impasse we aim for an even more rigid diet, increasing physical activity, with no result other than to make the situation worse.

Why does this happen? What are the mechanisms that are jammed and that make weight loss increasingly difficult despite the very little food consumed and the large amount of physical activity?
The answer is certainly not simple but a series of studies on the subject can give us important indications. This is a series of works that examine the production of cortisol in women, both

young and post-menopausal, subject to voluntary caloric restriction, which in everyday language is defined as diet.

Cortisol is a hormone that for years has had a bad press, like the colleague insulin, so much so that many of those pleasant popularizers who like to simplify have stuck on the label of hormone "bad". Nothing could be more wrong: the role of cortisol is crucial in regulating a whole series of body responses to variations in the surrounding and internal environment.

Cortisol is a glucocorticoid secreted by the adrenal glands, released in response to stress and reduction of blood glucose levels. Its role is to make available energy, mobilizing the stocks of sugars, proteins and fats, and at the same time to reduce the activities that could contribute to energy expenditure.

The activities on which cortisol has an inhibitory action are immune response, protein synthesis, DNA synthesis, production of growth hormone and testosterone. In practice, cortisol, in stressful situations, is released in order to make easily available a large amount of energy, necessary to cope with the stimulus that determined the secretion, diverting most of the resources of the organism for this purpose. So far nothing wrong, on the contrary, cortisol is a key element of the "fight or flight" mechanism so essential to our survival.

When the release of cortisol follows the normal daily pattern, with maximum in the morning, coinciding with the awakening, and minimum in the first hours of sleep, moment of rest and recovery, no problem. And no problem even when cortisol is released quickly in response to a stimulus, to then return, just as quickly, once the danger is overcome, to the basic levels.

Problems arise when cortisol levels become chronically elevated: under these conditions there is a marked catabolic effect, with progressive reduction of lean mass, an increase in fat mass, a consistently high blood sugar, loss of bone mass and an increase in fluid retention due to cortisol interactions with the mechanisms of elimination and reabsorption of sodium and potassium. Even short-term memory and sleep suffer greatly. It is in these conditions that cortisol becomes "bad", resulting in a series of unpleasant effects related to its continued secretion. If this situation continues for a long time the consequences can be very serious: it is not just about weight gain, but more susceptible to the metabolic syndrome and type 2 diabetes: all in all, it is worth trying to check better the production of this hormone.

Two important factors that may increase cortisol secretion are caloric restriction and exercise. That's right: being on a diet, especially when the diet is very strict and restrictive can lead to a rise in cortisol.

The relationship between diet is cortisol is well illustrated in the studies I mentioned in the initial part of the article. In all three studies, the diet of the subjects, young women in the first two, post-menopausal women in the third, was evaluated using the Three Factor Eating Questionnaire, a test that assesses the behavior of a person using three parameters:

voluntary caloric restriction, ie reduction of food intake in order to lose weight;
disinhibition, the tendency to consume food freely in response to specific stimuli, such as particular emotional states;
appetite, the tendency to consume food in response to physiological signals.
In the studies the subjects were divided into two groups according to their alimentary behavior: a group with strong voluntary caloric restriction, practically subject to diet, and a group with reduced caloric restriction, subjects with a normal

diet. To evaluate the daily secretion of cortisol, a urine collection was made in 24 hours, on a day in which the caloric intake was measured, taking care to keep the breakdown in macronutrients of the meals consumed constant, without any physical exercise and strictly in the first ten days following the cycle for young women, in order to minimize any confounding factors.

The results of the analyzes showed a marked increase in urinary excretion of cortisol, corresponding to a higher production, for subjects with greater caloric restriction; a result that goes to support the hypothesis that diet is an important stress factor able to determine an increase in cortisol secretion in 24 hours.

It should be noted that through the questionnaires it was possible to highlight how a rigid diet was often associated with an increase, also important, of physical exercise, often very intense. There are numerous studies that have shown that intense exercise can cause increased cortisol.

An additional factor that can contribute to worsening the problem is due to the progressive reduction of leptin that is observed during a diet. Leptin is a hormone produced by adipose tissue, able to modulate cortisol secretion. During a diet the production of leptin is reduced, therefore decreases its regulatory effect on the release of cortisol with further increase of the hormone, which is added to that caused by other factors.

In the end the data show clearly that a strict diet, especially when accompanied by too intense physical exercise, can contribute to a chronic elevation of cortisol, creating a situation that not only makes the sacrifices made vain, but also increases the risk of potential future problems, from osteoporosis to the metabolic syndrome.

Based on these studies, the conclusion to be drawn is not that diet and movement are a problem. Here we talk about dramatically restrictive diets, often with very low carbohydrate or protein content, and exasperated exercise: a type of behavior that is observed especially in young women, perhaps particularly worried about their physical fitness. An attitude to be avoided absolutely. Unfortunately, subjects with a certain profile to the contrary, when weight loss drops below their exaggerated expectations, they tend to further exacerbate caloric restriction and physical activity, eventually going to disturb their hormonal balance, with the end result of slowing down. until the loss of weight.

The solution to the problem is as simple as it is counterintuitive: loosen the grip of the diet a little, trying to increase the amount reserved for carbohydrates - of course quality, we do not talk about cookies, sweets and ice creams, but whole grains, pseudo-cereal as quinoa and buckwheat, legumes like chickpeas and lentils - and to take a little rest from physical activity: it often takes several days to improve the situation appreciably. Reducing the stress load resulting from controlled lifestyles can significantly contribute to refocusing the disturbed balance, bringing cortisol back to normal values.

Chapter 7: The importance of natural foods

There is a widespread belief, when it comes to food, that all that is natural is good and good, while any substance added, "chemistry" precisely, is unhealthy, dangerous and, in most cases, carcinogenic. The reality is different: in food there is in fact a large number of compounds, absolutely natural, which are potentially dangerous. Using as a risk indicator for a certain food the presence of "chemical" or "artificial" substances in opposition to the content of "natural" substances is therefore not particularly useful.

Often great attention is paid, and rightly so, to pesticides in food. Many studies have shown, however, that the content of natural pesticides, produced by the plant itself to protect itself against pests and predators, is definitely much higher than that of artificial pesticides, used in agricultural practice. Plants produce thousands of pesticide compounds, highly toxic and often carcinogenic. The classic study by Ames, Profet and Gold estimates that the daily intake of synthetic pesticides is about 0.09 mg, while that of natural pesticides averages around 1.5 g, thousands of times higher than the first.

Virtually more than 99% of the pesticides we consume with the diet are perfectly natural. The reason is simple: the plants have roots, they can not escape, and to defend themselves they can only produce toxic substances. Unfortunately, many of these substances, as well as for insects and other predators, are also toxic to humans and at least 60% have shown that they can cause cancer in rodents, obviously if given at much, much higher doses than those found in foods. Among these the Sinigrina, present in cabbage, broccoli and other brassicacce, the Estragolo present in fennel and basil, Safrolo in pepper, aniseed, nutmeg and parsley, but the list is very long.

This does not mean that fruits and vegetables can cause cancer by themselves, indeed all studies agree to underline the protective effect against these diseases, but shows that not all that is "natural" is good and indeed in many cases it can be very dangerous.

Plants and derivatives, even if completely natural, can be very dangerous when they are attacked by toxin-producing molds, which often occurs when storage and storage do not follow scrupulous hygiene and safety standards. Some molds that attack wheat, maize, peanuts can produce the fearsome aflatoxins, which can cause liver and esophagus cancer, as well as defects in fetal development.

The solanaceous produce the solanina, abundant above all in the potato, especially if the peel is greenish and rich in shoots, in the tomato and in the unripe aubergine. Toxin can cause severe gastric disorders, rarely hemorrhages, even more rarely death. Fortunately, its content is considerably reduced with maturation and cooking of the vegetables that contain it.

Furans are aromatic compounds with hepatic carcinogenic activity and may be present in olives, bread and especially in coffee, due to toasting, indeed it is estimated that coffee is the main source of exposure to furans.

The chemical risk ultimately reduces significantly in a varied diet, which can ward off dangerous accumulations of potentially harmful substances, natural or artificial; there is therefore no reason to be obsessed with the natural or "chemical" origin of the many compounds present in food.

Sometimes spasmodic attention is paid to the possible consumption of a few milligrams of synthetic substance, but the real danger of substances or foods consumed in quantity is neglected. Alcohol, for example, present in high quantities in many drinks usually consumed without any problem, is considered a carcinogenic substance for humans by the World Health Organization. Nitrosamines that are formed by cooking food, particularly frying, and nitrite and nitrate are also considered carcinogenic and even coffee is included among the potential causes of bladder tumors, although with an increase of very low risk.

In the end, if you look deeply, you will still find studies that show how ANY substance, natural or artificial, present in foods can be considered dangerous. However, individual studies must be interpreted in a broader context and often when they are examined comparing them with data related to several different works, certain correlations that seem very evident are significantly reduced.

Ultimately every food is nothing but a complex mixture of many different compounds: the artificial ones, which are added for the most different reasons, are subjected to a scrupulous evaluation of possible risks, with attention to both acute and chronic effects arising from exposure to these substances (to better understand how to evaluate the risk, read this article). Nothing can be considered completely safe and certainly it is necessary to carefully monitor the safety of artificial pesticides, additives and preservatives added to foods, limiting or blocking their use when data are available that give rise to even the slightest doubt.

Chapter 8: Paleo diet after the holidays

All happy and in company, we eat and drink, we celebrate, and, hopefully, we spend nice happy moments. The problems arrive in the following days, climbing on the scale, when, for many, the numbers are drawn upwards. But is it really so terrible what happened?
Party lunches are a social ritual for us Italians, a very important ritual to be lived in general in the family, a ritual for which we are willing to spend important amounts. It is a question, notwithstanding the different regional traditions, of very rich lunches in which the most daring can get to consume a significant amount of calories.

A quick count - span, without claim to absolute scientific accuracy - using the tools made available by sapermangiare.mobi (great site, full of useful information and tools: visit it!) Indicates that the average person can switch from a caloric intake daily about 2000-2500 kcal, at one of 4000-4500 kcal: a nice lunch with appetizer, two first courses, two second courses, side dishes, desserts, coffee and bitter. Maybe table heroes will be able to push themselves towards 6000 kcal, but also for them there is a physical limit to the capacity of food that can be consumed in a certain period of time.

If we talk about a single meal, at most two, probably the weight gain that we will see on the scale will be due only in part to an effective increase in body fat. One kg of fat contains about 9000 kcal. On a typical bank holiday you can consume maybe 3000-4000 kcal more than your daily requirement, corresponding to about 330-400g of fat: however not all these excess calories are actually converted into fat.

Firstly, there are studies that show how to consume a very large ration in a single meal, rather than in several meals during the day, determine an increase in the thermal effect of food. In short, the amount of energy dispersed in the form of heat is decidedly greater in the hours following the single, gargantuan meal, while it is more modest if the same calories are distributed in a certain number of smaller meals. In addition, studies on twin pairs of high-calorie diets for very long periods of time show that the accumulation of fat and the location of accumulated fat have a genetic basis: in fact, there were minimal variations in the fat accumulated by a pair of twins, important changes in that accumulated by different couples. Therefore, the role of genetics that governs the use of caloric surplus and type of accumulated tissue, fat or lean mass, seems significant.

The type of food that is actually consumed is also important. In the human body, part of the excess carbohydrates can be accumulated as glycogen in the liver and muscle. The quantity is not very relevant and can range from 300 to 500 g for an average individual. If large meals follow a period of intense training or consumption, the available glycogen stocks will be small and the body will use most of the carbohydrates consumed to restore these stocks: we are talking about 300-400 g of carbohydrates, a quantity certainly not despicable. Beyond the limit, part of the excess sugars will be used for the production of fats through lipogenesis processes.

The proteins present in food have a positive role: they reduce the appetite and stimulate heat production - again the thermal effect of food - so much so that several studies show that an increase in the daily caloric intake of some months, when the excess calories are due to the exclusive increase in protein, does not lead to a significant increase in body weight.

The problem arises when a significant proportion of excess comes from fats. These are substances that our body is very good to put aside and for which there is no limit to the ability to accumulate, so the more we find in the meal we consume the more we are susceptible to deposit it in adipose tissue. Same destiny for alcohol, and sparkling wines and wines never fail on the tables of the party: alcohol does not accumulate, of course, is burned to produce energy - and reduce toxicity to consumption - and by doing so allows the body to increase the share of sugars and fats to be allocated to the formation of adipose tissue. The cosmos conspires against us!

So, given that only a part of the nutrients present becomes fat and that the amount of fat deposited after a very abundant meal can not be of a kilo, how come, weighing the next morning, we find dammatic increases of one or two kg? Are we perhaps victims of tragic conspiracies?

I would say no, I suppose serious conspirators have better things to do than sabotage the scales on St. Stephen's morning, even if you can never say with certain conspirators. Much of the weight you see the day after is due to components that are NOT fat.

The first and most trivial is due to the glycogen stores, which after meals of this type are beautiful full. The problem is that one gram of glycogen carries around three grams of water, or even more, and that therefore for the accumulation of 300g of glycogen we must also consider the presence of 900 g of water to accompany it. And the first kilo is gone.

Other water you find in the bladder, so the advice is to weigh yourself after emptying it. And of course water and other material is in the intestine waiting to be recovered or eliminated. Even here, if your habits allow it, try to weigh yourself once "discharges". Total urine and faeces can contribute to over one kg of weight. And off with the second kilo.

Finally, body water can vary significantly depending on the consumption of salts, sugars and alcohol, certain medicines such as some antacids and physical activity, so even in this case we could observe also important changes. And the third kilo is gone.

In practice, most of the increase we see can be attributed to variations in the water content in different districts of the organism and only a small part can be due to the accumulation of fats. Remember that to be able to deposit only one kg of fat would require a caloric surplus of over 9000 kcal - probably much more - an amount that even the most gifted eaters have actually difficulty in swallowing.

The discourse is different if the excess is systematically repeated for several days, in which case the amount of fat deposited may eventually become significant: the increase in fat mass occurs over medium-long times. Otherwise, most of the increase recorded is due to the accumulation of salts and liquids.

Who does not love the binges is our microbiota, the lovely bacteria that are in our gut to work hard for our health in exchange for a hot meal. A caloric excess can alter the composition of the microbiota, especially when there is an important portion of refined carbohydrates, reducing the number of species present and favoring the development of species that can cause problems.

In the end the message is clear: one or two out-of-scale meals, in the economy of a healthy and varied diet, attentive to the real needs of the subject, can not create significant damage. The problem arises when the excessive consumption of food is sustained for long times.

Chapter 9: The importance of micronutrients

Not a day goes by without this or that substance in the media, obviously "chemistry", of synthesis, is described as a deadly danger, a cause of cancer and of infinite and mournful pathologies. The situation is much more complex than reported in the most bombastic and acchiappaclick titles. Not necessarily substances that are carcinogenic in the laboratory are in the real world, in vivo. And not all carcinogens are "chemical", indeed. This is what Bruce Ames, the man who designed the test that evaluates the ability of a substance to cause mutations and, therefore, cancer explains.

Bruce Ames is an American scientist, one of those old-fashioned, who has spent his career studying cancer and the factors that cause it. In the picture that portray him wearing the bow tie and a confident expression, evidence of a long career started in the 50s of the last century and dotted with important works, primarily the development of an effective test to determine the capacity of a substance to cause mutations.

Ames tells us that the idea was born by reading the list of ingredients on the potato chips he was eating. At that time Ames was studying some strains of Salmonella: it was almost spontaneous to wonder if those substances with the complicated name could cause mutations in its bacteria. So Ames developed a test to evaluate the mutagenicity of a given substance, using mutant strains of the bacteria that were the object of his studies.

The test designed by Ames is very quick and economical compared to long and expensive animal tests: using mice in general the first results are available after about three years.

Ames and colleagues, in the early 70s, used their test to evaluate a range of commonly used substances, and identified some of them - such as Tris BP (Tris [2,3-dibromopropyl] phosphate), a flame retardant used in the production of clothes for children, and AF 2 (Furilfuramide), a food additive widely used as a preservative in Japan - definitely dangerous and promptly eliminated from use. Ames became one of the first heroes of the environmental movement.

The hero's license was promptly withdrawn a few years later, when new work and statements by the scientist sparked fierce controversy.

Maybe that the good Ames is crazy, as sometimes happens to some luminary that maybe starts to deny the usefulness of the vaccines? It's not the case. The positions of the scientist are well argued and present very important points for reflection. Certainly an aid, to evaluate more critically and consciously many of the alarmist proclamations that so much hold on a public bewildered by constant and often unjustified alarms.

The structure of DNA is the same for all living things, so bacteria can be used to identify mutagens quickly, without having to wait months or years, as happens when they are used as mammalian guinea pigs, whose life cycle is very , much longer than that of a microorganism: two or three years for a mouse versus twenty minutes for a bacterium. The Ames test uses different strains of Salmonella typhimurium, carriers of mutations in a gene that encodes a protein involved in the synthesis of histidine, an amino acid. Because of these mutations the bacteria are not able to grow in culture media without this compound: they are auxotrophic for histidine, as they say in scientific jargon.

These bacteria are grown in soils containing progressively increasing doses of the test substance and a small amount of histidine, which allows the initial growth of the colonies and therefore the opportunity to generate mutants. Some of these mutants will be revertants: due to mutations they will again acquire the ability to synthesize histidine and may still grow, despite the absence of the amino acid in the culture medium. In practice we will have a reduced or no bacterial growth if the substance tested is not a mutagen, while the growth will be significant, with the formation of numerous colonies, when the test substance is able to induce mutations.

Tested on known mutagens, the test managed to identify 70-90%: it is therefore a useful tool to identify new ones. To better simulate the conditions that are observed in vivo, in mammals, an extract of rat liver enzymes is added to the culture medium: some substances are not mutagenic by themselves, but can become by the detoxification enzymes present in the 'body.

In most tests the dose / response effect is almost always linear: a result that suggests that there is no safety threshold, a concentration of the substance below which there is no mutagenesis. However, Ames pointed out that at very low concentrations of mutagen, those that actually occur in vivo, the role of DNA repair mechanisms becomes important, since they can eliminate mutations as they are formed; moreover, part of the effects observed at the high concentrations used in the test may not actually be due to the mutagenic action of the compounds, but to their mitogenetic action, ie their ability to stimulate bacterial division.

It should be emphasized that the mutagens identified with this test do not necessarily need to be considered carcinogenic: this is a first step requiring accurate subsequent evaluations with eukaryotic cell tests and in vivo animal studies. However, there is a strong correlation between the mutagenic effects detected through the Ames test and the actual carcinogenicity in humans.

The Ames test is a milestone in research but the good doctor has certainly not rested on his laurels and, after having introduced and perfected the test, he has worked on the topic for a long time. His studies on the role that free radicals have in causing mutations, in the genesis of numerous degenerative diseases and in aging are very interesting. And even more interesting is his study of the early '90s in which he examined the nature and quantity of a large number of substances present in fruit and vegetables, not limited to synthetic products but also investigating the substances naturally present in plants.

In the Ames study, he pointed out that only a small part of these natural pesticides present in plants was subjected to the Ames test, just over fifty, and that of these over 50% was mutagenic at high concentrations, a very similar percentage to those of the tested synthesis substances.

Ultimately according to Ames the amount of pesticides and pollutants that we consume with the diet is very much reduced compared to the huge amount of naturally occurring substances in food. And an additional quota of potentially dangerous substances is formed during cooking, another 2 grams of compounds, some of which are carcinogenic to the Ames test or on mice: polycyclic hydrocarbons, heterocyclic amines and nitrosamines.

Ames takes coffee as an example, one of the most consumed beverages in the world. A single cup - presumably American, therefore plentiful - contains about 10 mg of mutagenic compounds in the Ames test and identified as carcinogens in animal tests: a quantity equal to one third of the total sum of synthetic pesticides assumed in a year through the foods.

Ames emphasizes that our body has tools that are able to counteract the effects of these substances. These tools are not specific but general, given the enormous amount of toxic compounds with which man has had to do during the evolution: the cells of those parts of the body that come into contact with these substances are continually eliminated and replaced , from the skin to the mucous membranes of the digestive and respiratory system; the cells exposed to the action of mutagens and oxidants develop strong defenses against them; the liver works actively for the detoxification and excretion of these compounds; finally, at the DNA level, repair mechanisms are active to eliminate errors due to the action of mutagens. These are therefore effective mechanisms both for toxins present in plants and for synthetic compounds.

Obviously Ames certainly does not mean that consuming coffee or vegetables is carcinogenic or that we can spray with herbicides with joy our garden. The conclusion of Ames is that exposure to these synthetic compounds - even when these substances are positive for Ames test or animal studies - is a negligible factor in the genesis of cancer, when compared to the much more important exposure to mutagenic substances naturally present in food, to those that are formed during cooking or to those inhaled by smokers.

According to Ames, the main causes of cancer are mutagenesis, DNA damage, and mitogenesis or stimulation of cell division. Mutagenic substances produce DNA damage that causes cells to divide without control. Obviously, a number of mutations are required before a normal cell turns into a tumor cell and begins to proliferate uncontrollably. It is natural to think that all mutagens are external substances - chemicals, as many people like to call them - but in reality a large part of these mutagens are produced in our body, during normal metabolic processes, particularly at the mitochondria level, the energy cell: it is precisely in these organelles that a significant share of free radicals is formed, aggressive substances capable of producing significant damage at the DNA level. Therefore, the respiratory processes that take place in the cell produce most of the problems: Ames calculates that in one day about 10,000 oxidative damage can occur to the DNA of every single cell. Obviously these damages are promptly repaired by very efficient, but not perfect, mechanisms: over time, the damage tends to accumulate and are added to those charged with proteins and lipids, still due to the action of free radicals.

The presence of these damages at the DNA level translates into mutations when the cell divides. Cells with a high rate of division are likely to become cancerous cells more easily than those that are less frequently divided. All agents that stimulate cell division must therefore be considered risk factors: estrogens, which cause proliferation in the cells of the breast; hepatitis B and C viruses and alcohol, which cause lesions in the liver and thus proliferation of the liver cells to reduce the damage; a high consumption of salt or Helicobacter infections responsible for inflammation of the stomach mucosa; the papilloma virus that induces cell proliferation of the cervix; asbestos or tobacco smoke that irritate the lung areas and tissues. For many of the chemicals identified as carcinogenic, the usual exposure must be very close to the toxic dose, because the effect may be significant: a condition that is generally observed in those who daily handle large quantities of these compounds for work. However, at these concentrations, more than the mutagenic effect prevails a real cytotoxic effect, with extensive lesions affecting different cellular components.

Ames points out that the incidence of cancer increases significantly with age: it is therefore a degenerative disease linked to aging. External factors can increase the risk, such as smoking in humans, or reduce it, for example the caloric restriction in rodents, today so studied. Surely, a major factor in determining risk is the basal metabolism: the higher this is, the greater is the production of free radicals, so important in determining lesions at the DNA level.

Ames believes there may be a lack of vitamins and minerals among the causes of cancer. These micronutrients are essential to maintain a high efficiency of mitochondria and cell repair processes, with a significant reduction in the risk of mutagenesis. In this regard, Ames has proposed the theory of triage, according to which, in the case of lack of these micronutrients - a very frequent event in our evolutionary history - the body tends to use the reduced amounts available for those critical processes necessary for survival in short term. Under these conditions, all those activities that are responsible for long-term survival are penalized, including those of DNA repair mechanisms, essential to prevent mutations, and of oxidative lesions on proteins and lipids.

Among the micronutrients studied by Ames we have magnesium, vitamin D, vitamin K, selenium, zinc, vitamin B12, folate, iron. The deficiency of each of these substances forces the body to make difficult choices, diverting the minimum quantities available of the nutrient to the activities necessary for immediate survival, to the detriment of those processes that are essential to maintain the integrity of mitochondria and DNA.

Ames therefore concludes that the lack of these micronutrients, a probably more widespread problem than we think, can be dangerous for our health, a risk factor for cancer much more important than the small amount of pesticides that may be present in fruit and vegetables.

Bruce Ames is a biochemist. A researcher with a splendid career, but still a single voice. The opinion of an expert is only a personal opinion, certainly it is the opinion of those who study the topic from a lifetime but, as I wrote in another article, has no scientific value if not supported by data. And on the subject Ames brings interesting data, with his scientific works.

Certainly its position on pesticides and pollutants may appear out of tune with respect to the prevailing chorus in the media, but it is important to reflect.

Unfortunately, they are generally the themes of little importance but of sure media grip to capture the attention of the public. We eat too much, we eat badly, but we are worried about the infinitesimal traces of some chemical compound in our wine. Traces thousands of times below the risk threshold. While of alcohol, a carcinogen of class 1, dozens of grams are thrown down every day.

Ames has never worked for the industry, nor did he provide advice or expertise for companies. He does not publish books, he does not go on television, he does not sell diets of immortality, detoxifying or regenerating. He is a scientist who does his job. Observe, hypothesis advances, experimentally test, verify if the data support hypotheses. And from the numbers and the data draws conclusions.

In the end, his advice is trivial: eat more vegetables and more fruit, keep fit and be active. Put your body in a position to work to the best of its ability, provide micronutrients, vitamins and minerals here, so important for the efficiency of our repair and defense mechanisms against the ravages of time, breathing, contaminants and other foreign substances . Concentrate on improving your diet and lifestyle and pay less attention to details that, all things considered, are irrelevant.

Chapter 10: The best paleo food – pomegranate

A symbol of fertility, present in ancient myths, the pomegranate is a fruit with remarkable nutritional properties, rich in antioxidants, a real panacea for health, with its crimson beans with a sweet, acidic and astringent taste.
The pomegranate is the fruit of a bushy tree, Punica Granatum, which grows very well in arid and poor soils, with cold winters and very hot summers. The plant is native to the fertile crescent, between the Mediterranean and the Middle East, and was already appreciated and widespread among the Egyptians and the ancient Babylonians. Always a symbol of fertility, due to the large number of seeds produced, a prominent place had in the Greek myths: it was a pomegranate the fruit that Ade used to tempt Proserpina and take her as a bride in the underworld.
Much widespread and appreciated until 1800, its consumption as a fresh fruit has decreased considerably, although in recent years has known a new popularity in the form of juice with amazing nutritional properties.
Currently the main producers are Iran, India and the United States, but in our gardens it is not rare to find robust plants that are loaded with ripe red fruits in autumn.

The plant can grow up to 8 meters in height, but is generally kept low and bushy. The spring flowers, red and large, give rise to fruits that are harvested ready for consumption as the maturation stops when they are detached from the plant.

The fruits, which from the botanical point of view are berries, have a very thick and hard peel, rich in tannins, red for most varieties. Inside a white membrane, also very rich in astringent compounds, draws different sections in which the seeds nest, from 200 to 1500 per fruit, surrounded by a bright red pulp, sweet when fully ripe, with a remarkable level of acidity and strong astringent notes due to the high content of tannins.

In recent years the pomegranate has returned to the limelight, after years of obscure arbitrary, thanks to its significant nutritional properties: 100 grams of grains give about 80 kcal with a fat content of just over a gram, of proteins around two grams and of carbohydrates of about 19 grams, of which 4 grams of fiber and 15 grams of sugars, essentially sucrose, fructose and glucose. Good content of potassium, copper, manganese and phosphorus. Vitamin C, vitamin K and folate also abound. Abundant organic acids in species citric acid. What makes the pomegranate a superfood, as the American enthusiasts like to say, is the relevant content in polyphenols, phytonutrients which, among other things, give the typical red color, abundant in fruits but even more in the rind that is in fact raw material for the extraction of these principles, used in the production of food supplements. Among the polyphenols present, in addition to the tannins responsible for the astringent taste, also ellagitannins or punicalagus, large molecules formed by the union between ellagic acids and carbohydrates, which can however be absorbed at the intestinal level. In the seeds there is a particular polyunsaturated fatty acid, the punicic acid, which is also widely studied.

The pomegranate should be picked or bought well ripe. The fruits must have a dark red rind, compact and free of dents, and must be heavy and solid. Avoid those with wrinkled, opaque, discolored and stained peel.
The pomegranate, you will have noticed, is very difficult to open: you have to have strong nerves and cut slowly to prevent the crimson juice from the grains splash everywhere transforming the bystanders in many extras of horror movies.

The grains are delicious eaten naturally, especially if the fruit is at the right degree of ripeness, but can be used in the most disparate recipes.

The red and juicy grains are excellent ingredients for salads, with rocket or spinach for example, for a pleasant contrast of flavors between the bitter touch of the leaves and the release of the sweet and sour juice of the beans. Excellent risottos, with the juice that can be used for cooking rice, giving an aroma that goes well with experimenting with vegetable creams. Extraordinary meat dishes, where juice and beans give color and flavor the most varied cuts and meats.

In the oriental kitchen the pomegranate is a basic ingredient for the most varied dishes: the powder of pomegranate seeds is a much appreciated spice, anardana, in India and Pakistan, while beans, molasses juice and pomegranate are present in many recipes of the kitchen Iranian.

Grenadine is the syrup made from the boiling of pomegranate juice, a non-alcoholic drink, once very widespread, used both for the preparation of granite and for the preparation of cocktails and long drinks such as Shirley Temple or Tequila Sunrise. On the market there is granatina also obtained from citrus fruits, currants, raspberries or aromas. You, drinkers with a refined palate, be wary of these pale imitations.

The antioxidant potential of the pomegranate is superior to that of green tea and red wine. For this reason, in recent years, the pomegranate has become the subject of a large number of studies with results of considerable practical interest. The focus was mainly on the search for positive effects related to the consumption of juice, rich in punicalagin, and the oily extract of the seeds, where the punicic acid abounds.

In vivo and in vitro studies have shown a protective effect against various forms of cancer. The juice has been used in studies on patients with prostate cancer whose growth seems to be slowing down significantly.

In the laboratory, fermented juice showed a strong antiproliferative effect on breast tumors. A chemo-protective effect has also been recorded for lung, colon and skin cancers. An important result of these studies, which are all at the preliminary stage, has been to highlight that the effect of the juice is greater than that of the single purified substances, a fact that underlines the synergistic effect of the large quantity of compounds present in the fruit, each of which probably acts at different levels contributing to an overall result that is decidedly higher than the sum of the parts.

The consumption of pomegranate juice can reduce blood pressure, can reduce the formation of atherosclerotic plaque and the peroxidation of lipids that contributes to this process, with a reduction of LDL cholesterol and an increase in HDL; a series of effects that reasonably suppose a significant protective effect on the cardiovascular system.

In vitro and animal studies have also shown that the antioxidant and anti-inflammatory activity of pomegranate juice can help reduce the problems related to osteoarthritis and rheumatoid arthritis, by intervening on the main mediators of inflammatory and degenerative processes.

In diabetic subjects, pomegranate juice has been shown to increase insulin sensitivity while significantly reducing oxidative stress related to the disease.

Even the extract of pomegranate flowers has shown remarkable virtues. In some studies on obese subjects its use was associated with a reduction in weight and fat tissue and a reduction in blood sugar, HDL cholesterol and triglycerides.

Pomegranate juice has strong antimicrobial and fungicidal activity: results in the laboratory against Candida Albicans, against resistant antibiotic strains of Staphylococcus aureus and against enterohemorrhagic cepi of Escherichia coli.

There are also studies that have evaluated the effect of pomegranate juice on male erectile dysfunction: the results seem encouraging, but further studies on the topic are required before reaching conclusive data.

At the current state of the studies, the consumption of pomegranate juice or extracts and concentrates does not present any side effects, even for very high concentrations of the most important active ingredients. Some studies are under way to determine potential drug interactions: pomegranate juice may interfere with cytochrome C450, the liver enzyme responsible for the metabolism of a large number of drugs, even if the work available has shown appreciable effects. However, if you take anticoagulants or benzodiazepines, avoid consuming large amounts of juice to keep yourself safe.

A plant that grows in difficult conditions, an ancient fruit mentioned in myths and legends, brightly colored grains and sweet and pungent taste, suitable for different and tasty recipes, a juice with great preventive and even therapeutic properties: I would say that there are reasons to consume more often this fruit there are really.

Chapter 11: The problem with nutritional studies

Not a day goes by without the stupefying results of dozens of scientific studies on nutrition bouncing on the media. Results that perhaps contradict the data published only a short time before or even overturn those that seemed positions now acquired. A fact that creates disorientation and confusion, fueling doubts and fears that often leave room for those on speculating and prosperous fears and hopes.

Scrolling through the media reports of scientific research in the field of nutrition is legitimate to try a little confusion: before saturated fats are evil and should be avoided like the plague, then it is the turn of carbohydrates that are solely responsible for the current epidemic of obesity; mindful of the proteins that destroy the kidneys, but if you are elderly, increase their consumption; the meat causes cancer, but not all, only the preserved one; fish is good, but better to avoid containing mercury; the eggs inexorably increase cholesterol, no, they are fine! And so on, in a whirlwind of different indications, often conflicting, that obviously leave the disoriented and doubtful non-professionals, creating situations that allow the prospering of a whole undergrowth of subjects that make strong of this or that data, often selected and manipulated to art, they propose pseudoscientific solutions so imaginative and ineffective as suggestive, however always very advantageous (economically) for those who propose them.

Why in the field of nutrition is this noticeable variability of indications, this reversal of positions that seemed very solid and then turned out to be exaggerated or even contradicted? Why even scientific studies - letting the media lose, that they must do with rebellious titles - very often give radically different results that make it difficult to unequivocally clarify issues of great interest, starting from the role of specific nutrients in the genesis of specific diseases?

The answer is not simple: there are many factors that contribute to determining this situation, factors that depend both on the complexity of the themes studied, both on the ways in which these issues are investigated, and on the techniques used to analyze the results.

Studying the impact that the consumption of a given food has on our health is not easy. The effects of the consumption of a given food are not immediate, often revealed after years or tens of years. Therefore, very long and very complex studies are needed because as well as time it is also necessary to take into account the impact of a whole series of other factors that could significantly contribute to determining the observed results. Many of the studies that seek to clarify how specific nutrients can affect our health are cohort studies, jobs that follow large groups of people for long periods, gathering a large number of information related to different variables, such as consumption of certain foods, styles of life, physical activity and so on. After a certain period of time some characteristics of the group examined are compared to control groups, often the population as a whole, in order to test specific hypotheses. In this type of work the selection of the subjects studied, the parameters considered, the way in which the information is collected, the techniques with which they are elaborated, can significantly influence the final results: studies with similar objectives but with significant differences related to indicated criteria can give different results.

Obviously all these factors are clearly indicated and taken into consideration by those who study it, so the results are always interpreted with some caution. However, the possibility remains that many of the observed effects may be due to particular factors linked to the lifestyle of the subjects studied or to other factors not taken into consideration. A small example: a series of cohort studies performed on members of the Adventist, vegetarian or semi-vegetarian sect for religious reasons, has shown that a vegetarian diet involves a reduction of mortality from all causes, particularly for cardiovascular diseases, with more important among men. These are interesting data, but the authors of the works are the first to point out that the studied group is very particular, has a different life style from that of the general population, with very low alcohol consumption, greater physical activity and strong social cohesion. which the effects observed could be attributable to the contribution of various factors and not only to the parameters considered. Work examining more homogeneous groups, for example vegan and omnivorous subjects with similar attention to diet composition and lifestyle in general, do not show significant differences between the two groups, both characterized by a lower mortality compared to the general population : data that seem to indicate that the protective role observed, rather than being ascribable to the consumption of specific foods, is in reality due to the lifestyle as a whole.

Clinical studies are also not without problems: in these works subjects are randomly assigned to two groups, one of which is subjected to a specific intervention while the other is used as a control group. The random assignment to the two groups is aimed at reducing the possibility of distortions due to the selection of subjects or the specific modalities of the study, and increase the probability that the differences are actually due to the treatment used. Studies of this type are, as you can imagine, very complex and expensive to implement, often the number of participants is reduced, often particular populations are investigated - for example obese or diabetic subjects - often the survey is performed for limited periods of time, many times the operation is done using the quantity and mode of consumption of the food that are decidedly far from those usually done in everyday life. The difficulties are there both when investigating the effect on health due to the consumption of a nutrient and that one intends to evaluate what happens what happens when consumption is instead decreased. If I reduce the consumption of saturated fats in the diet but at the same time increases the consumption of other nutrients the observed effect is due to the reduction of the first or the increase of the second? Many times it is not so simple to understand it and the final result of the work can vary in an important way, even if the survey concerns the same theme, depending on the specific intervention modalities of the different works.

And indeed, while the media like to relaunch the results of individual studies with emphatic tones, in the scientific field studies, from preliminary work on cell cultures or on the animal model to population or clinical studies, are only single pieces of a puzzle that the professional prepared can be very complex, composed of thousands of different pieces, to be put together with great patience and attention. In fact, an important role has systematic reviews and meta-analyzes, works that examine and re-elaborate the results of the studies available on a specific topic, so as to arrive at conclusions that take into account all the factors that, as we have seen, can help to determine very different results. It is on the basis of this type of work that the indications and guidelines of the various organizations dealing with health are elaborated. And as you can often guess, works of this kind do not come to clear conclusions, in black and white, but indicate potential, probability, nuances that depend in fact on many different factors and not on a single element.

Of course, it would be easier if the research could unequivocally indicate that a certain food is the cause of every evil while another is the cure of every affliction, but science does not work like that, and in particular it does not work that science investigates the issues related to health and nutrition, a sector in which the variables that can influence the results of the observations are many, and often difficult to evaluate.

I certainly do not mean to discredit the precious, precious and difficult work of those who investigate certain topics, essential to enable us to clarify, one piece at a time, the relationship that exists between nutrition, lifestyle and health. What I want to emphasize is that if the results may appear to be conflicting and generate confusion it is not because the studies are worthless or manipulated: they are the complexity of the subject, the large number of parameters to be considered, the difficulty in assessing the real impact of specific intervention, to determine the lack of homogeneity of the results. Unevenness that those working in this area try to overcome by refining the tools used in order to progressively reduce the disturbing factors capable of polluting the data collected.

The scientific investigation is a process in continuous evolution, a constant revision and elaboration of the models in the light of the collected data, a work that does not produce a definitive and monolithic truth but a set of knowledge that are the result of this continuous work of study. So when we read of the amazing results of a certain work, perhaps presented using stereotyped statements of the tenor of "Science says" (with capital letters, I recommend), we try not to be carried away by enthusiasm and we evaluate carefully, critically and objective, what we are told, whether we confirm what we knew - or we thought we knew - that it contradicts it, a situation that instead of confusing or infuriating us, as often happens, should push us to reflect on the topic, deepening all the aspects without stop at the surface as often happens.

Chapter 12: Another great paleo food – kiwi

In the 70s, when it appeared for the first time in Italy, the kiwi was presented as the fruit of health; and for once the advertising did not exaggerate, given the remarkable nutritional properties of this fruit originating in China but selected and baptized in the distant New Zealand.

The Kiwi plant is native to China, where it was mainly used for ornamental purposes. The fortune of the fruit begins in the early 1900s, when Isabel Fraser, returning from a visit to China, brought some seeds with her in her native New Zealand. The plant must have intrigued local farmers, especially Hayward Wright, who selected the most cultivated variety, the Hayward, by planting the first orchards for large-scale production in the 30s.

The cultivation of kiwi at the beginning was difficult but the many problems to be addressed did not prevent its spread, first in nearby Australia, then in the Americas and finally in Europe. The name of the fruit, inspired by the Kiwi bird, symbol of New Zealand, was proposed by Turners & Grovers, an export company in Auckland, and met immediate success.

Currently the world's largest producer of kiwis is China, the country of origin, followed by Italy, which with its 523,000 tons per year also surpassed New Zealand in the late 80s. The Italian was a success obtained using simple means but effective to recreate the microclimate necessary for the development of the plant, with abundant shade obtained using nets and nebulization of water between the leaves to keep them constantly humid.

The kiwi fruit is an oval berry that has very different sizes and colors depending on the species and varieties considered. The Hayward, the most common cultivar, belongs to the Actinidia deliciosa species and has large, egg-shaped fruits with hairy peel and green pulp characterized by the presence of a crown of black seeds arranged around a central portion of lighter vascular tissue. The taste of ripe fruit is sugary and slightly acidic with hints of flowers and herbs due to the abundant presence of volatile compounds, esters, alcohol and aldehydes

The other commonly cultivated species is Actinidia chinensis, which has a smooth and bronzed skin and golden pulp that has earned it the name of kiwi gold or Zespri. The fruit can also be consumed without removing the peel, given the absence of hair, and has a sweeter taste and even richer in aromas than the Hayward, very similar to that of other tropical fruits.

Other species, Actinidia arguta, Actinidia kolomitka and Actinidia polygama, give small berries, with smooth and thin skin and a taste very similar to that of green kiwi, and have a very limited commercial diffusion.

The kiwi plant is a vine that, like the vine, gives long and flexible branches that need support, with female plants and male plants. Pollination in the wild is the work of birds and insects and is difficult to obtain because the flowers are not particularly attractive to bees. Therefore, saturation pollination techniques are used, with a large number of beehives per hectare of orchard, a situation that forces insects to also use kiwi flowers due to the intense competition for flowers available at a distance of flight.

The plant loves the shade and neutral or acid soils while it does not tolerate calcareous soils, the environment must be damp, irrigation is necessary only if the soil becomes dry, more importantly reduce the loss of water through the leaves, shading the plant with nets and spraying water between the leaves. Fertilizers with nitrogen, phosphorus and potassium are necessary to give numerous, large and succulent fruits.

The plant begins to produce after about a year and remains productive for about ten years. Pruning is very important and allows you to maintain a good productivity over time, with the branches older than three years that must be eliminated because they no longer bear fruit.

The plant is very sensitive to stagnant water, can be attacked by aphids and cochineals, bacteria and fungi that reduce its production capacity and can cause significant economic damage if not properly treated.

In Italy kiwifruit is harvested from November, harvesting is done by hand when the fruits are still hard and still. The kiwi fruit is a climacteric fruit that continues to ripen even after harvesting: the process can be stopped by keeping the fruits well chilled and in complete absence of ethylene, a gas that in plants acts as a hormone and promotes the ripening of the fruit. Bananas, apples and pears are great producers of ethylene and particularly hard kiwis can be quickly matured by placing them in a closed container together with some of these fruits.

Italian production does not overlap with that of Chile and New Zealand and this makes the fruit available throughout the year.

A typical kiwi, a fruit weighing about 75 grams, gives a contribution of 46 kcal. Most of these come from sugars, about 11 grams. In the still unripe fruit a good part of these sugars is in the form of starch but during the maturation conversion into simple sugars, especially glucose and fructose in almost equal quantities, about 3 grams each, with small amounts of residual sucrose. The fibers are very abundant, about 2, 5 grams, and are represented by polysaccharides of the cell walls: pectins for the soluble portion, cellulose and hemicellulose for the insoluble portion. Fats and proteins are present in small amounts, just one gram each. Vitamin C, E, K and folate are very abundant, potassium, calcium and magnesium are good.

The kiwi is rich in chlorophyll, which gives the typical green color to the pulp and that in some varieties, with yellow, red or violet pulp, is reduced during maturation with a marked increase in carotenoids such as lutein, zeaxanthin and β-carotene. There are also significant quantities of secondary metabolites such as caffeic acid, quinic acid, chlorogenic acid, flavones and flavonones, substances with a strong antioxidant action.

Among the proteins present, actinidine, an enzyme that attacks proteins, and kiwellin, is particularly important. During the maturation after harvesting, by act of actinidine, it forms some biologically active peptides such as kissper and KiTh.

The kiwi arrived in Italy in the 70s. The first communication campaigns to promote consumption presented it as the "fruit of health" and for once the advertising hyperbole was not so far from the truth: the kiwi is in fact a very rich food of important nutrients and its regular consumption can really bring health benefits.

The kiwi is very rich in vitamin C, a single fruit can meet the daily requirement, with a slightly higher intake for the yellow pulp variant. Vitamin C is an important antioxidant, it is essential for a good functionality of the immune system and favors the absorption of iron present in food. Consumption of a single kiwifruit per day allows to reach what is considered the optimal concentration of vitamin C in plasma and tissues, with full saturation already with the consumption of only two fruits per day.

The kiwi also has a good content of vitamin E, another precious compound with antioxidant action, and folate: the latter also abound in green leafy vegetables, but are easily degraded during cooking, so a good consumption of the fruit can contribute to a adequate supply of these precious substances.

Other micronutrient present in large quantities is potassium: a constant consumption of the fruit can contribute to maintaining a good Na + / K + ratio, a ratio that many studies have shown to be decisively important in reducing the risk of hypertension and cardiovascular diseases

Next to vitamin C and vitamin E there is a large number of antioxidant substances, most of which have been stable and well absorbed in the intestine. Several studies have shown that a constant consumption of kiwi can improve some parameters related to inflammatory processes and cardiovascular diseases, with a significant increase in the level of HDL cholesterol.

Interesting studies have shown that consumption of a single kiwifruit after the evening meal can improve the quality of sleep, reducing the time needed to fall asleep and the time needed to wake up; these are preliminary works that nevertheless indicate interesting fields of study.

Kiwi consumption, thanks to the abundant fiber content, can contribute to modify the intestinal microbiota, favoring the short-term increase of lactobacilli and bifidobacteria. These variations in the microbiota and the strong affinity of the fruit fibers for liquids - which leads to a large increase in the volume of faecal material - may be among the factors that give kiwifruit a laxative action. Also the actinidine and kiwilleine present in the fruit, enzymes able to hydrolyse proteins, could help to make gastric emptying faster and promote intestinal motility. From the kiwellin derives the kissper peptide which is resistant to the action of proteolytic enzymes and therefore remains functional in the intestine where it exerts an important anti-inflammatory action while favoring the secretion of liquids in the intestinal lumen. Thanks to the good relationship between glucose and fructose and the reduced content of fructans, kiwi can also be consumed by subjects who have altered sensitivity to FODMAP, on the contrary, it can become a valuable ally to reduce constipation in those individuals with irritable bowel syndrome accompanied by stubborn constipation.

Unfortunately, the kiwi also presents numerous allergens, first of all actinidine, which in sensitive individuals can give manifestations that can also be very severe, especially in children. People suffering from latex allergy can have cross-reactivity with kiwi and therefore should consume the fruit with extreme care.

The kiwi is harvested still hard and the ripening can be completed by keeping the fruit at room temperature or, if very hard, in a closed container with some apples. The kiwi is ready for consumption when the pulp is slightly yielding to the pressure of the fingers. Discard fruits that are too soft or bruised, excessively ripe and have an unpleasant taste. At room temperature, the kiwi can be stored for a few days, while in the refrigerator, if it is very hard, it can last for two or three weeks.

The kiwi is very good eaten naturally: a well-ripened fruit is rich in taste and aroma. Even the peel is edible and the gold varieties, with a smooth skin, are often eaten without being peeled. The kiwi goes well with fruit salads, sorbets, cereals, cakes, ice cream and yogurt. In the fruit salads it is good to add the kiwi shortly before consumption, to avoid that the enzymes present make the other fruits soft. Even in milk-based products it is good to add the kiwi at the last moment or after having scalded it, to avoid that the enzymes present can curdle the milk. Enzymes that can instead be used to make the meat more tender, simply rubbing a slice of fresh kiwi on the surface of the meat and letting it rest for about twenty minutes.

The kiwi can be blended or squeezed to obtain its juice: in both cases it is advisable to avoid excessive pressures that can crush the small seeds, since their content can give an unpleasant bitter taste to the product. The kiwi can also be cooked, even fried, always taking care not to overly treat it, to avoid losing its aroma and freshness.

Chapter 13: Is low carb a good alternative to the paleo diet?

Maintaining the weight achieved after a weight loss diet is difficult for many people and the strategies used to avoid recovering the lost kilos are many. A study published in The British Medical Journal indicates a possible strategy, effective especially for certain subjects: follow a low-carb diet.

Any diet is always accompanied by some physiological adaptations that reduce its effectiveness over time. Among these it is hypothesized that the progressive reduction of energy expenditure that would be caused by the limited caloric intake can play an important role. It would also increase the feeling of hunger, creating a situation that for many subjects makes it really difficult to maintain the weight achieved thanks to the diet.

To explain this situation some authors hypothesize that it is the consumption of increasing amounts of carbohydrates - especially simple sugars, which cause a strong release of insulin - to promote the accumulation of nutrients consumed in the adipose tissue, with consequent increase in weight and of fat mass. In these conditions, hunger would be increased and energy expenditure decreased and then a correct weight would be increasingly difficult to maintain. A model that has often been questioned, with some recent meta-analyzes that do not seem to show significant differences in energy expenditure between subjects that follow low-carb and low-fat diets.

A recent study published in "The British Medical Journal" shows a different picture, definitely in favor of low-carb diets. And since this is a clinical study with a very interesting protocol it is worth examining the results carefully.

The main authors of the "Effects of a low carbohydrate diet" study are Ebbeling and Ludwig, both of Harvard Medical School in Boston. Ludwig in particular is one of the main proponents of the theory that sees the binomial carbohydrate-insulin as the main responsible for what is now considered a veritable epidemic of obesity.

The study recruited 234 overweight and obese subjects who in a first phase followed a basic diet - 45% carbohydrate nutrient breakdown, 30% fat, 25% protein - for about 10 weeks. Those who have lost at least 12% of their initial weight, a weight loss that is characteristic of most of the commonly used diets, have been recruited for the second phase of the work.

The 162 subjects who had a satisfactory weight loss were assigned, in a completely random manner, to three different groups, each of which followed a maintenance diet with different carbohydrate content:

high carbohydrate diet, 60% of total calories
medium carbohydrate diet, 40% of total calories
low carbohydrate diet, 20% of total calories
120 subjects completed the course, which lasted 20 weeks, maintaining the weight reached at the end of the slimming phase, with maximum oscillations of about 2 kg.

For each subject different parameters were evaluated, with measurements related to energy expenditure, glucose concentration, insulin, ghrelin and leptin, using very precise techniques. The subjects have eaten meals specially prepared for each of them, in order to eliminate potential disturbing factors, inevitably present when a person prepares his own food in an autonomous way.

The results of the work show some interesting points:

Total energy expenditure is higher in subjects with a low-carb diet, with a difference between 209 and 278 kcal per day. In practice, a decrease in total energy expenditure of around 50-70 kcal / day is observed for a 10% increase in the contribution of carbohydrates to the total caloric intake. An effect that has not been reduced during the 20 weeks of surgery and which could therefore be directly linked to the breakdown of diet macronutrients. The authors have calculated that a similar effect could lead to losing about 10 kg in three years, given that the subject does not significantly change his diet;
The levels of ghrelin are lower in subjects with low-carb diets. Ghrelin is a hormone produced by the stomach and pancreas that increases the sensation of hunger, thus leading to greater consumption of food, reduces energy expenditure and promotes the accumulation of fatty tissue;
Leptin levels are lower in subjects with a low-carb diet. Leptin is produced by adipose tissue and a reduction in this case seems to suggest an increase in sensitivity to the action of this hormone - which is among those responsible for the feeling of satiety - as evidenced by some epidemiological studies that showed a greater decline of leptin levels after a diet involves a lower risk of recovery of lost weight.
An important fact that emerges from the study is that these effects are much greater in those subjects that present a greater secretion of insulin, a fact that seems to suggest that in particular populations the composition of the maintenance diet can play a very important role in the success long-term diet.

Strengths of the study are the strict control over the participants, which has made it possible to eliminate many disturbing factors, careful control over the composition of the diet followed in both phases, the use of very precise measurement techniques and the long duration of the 'intervention.

There remains the risk that, despite very precise measurement techniques, there are still errors in the assessment of total energy expenditure, and that there may have been transgressions of those who, although receiving personalized meals, are not monitored constantly and may have transgressed, even if Data analysis techniques have tried to take into account these factors and other potential disturbances such as the level of physical activity, the thermal effect of the foods consumed and the activity of brown adipose tissue.

Ultimately, the study indicates that in the medium term, a low-carb diet allows to easily maintain the weight achieved after a weight-loss diet, particularly in those subjects who at the beginning of the weight-loss process have a greater secretion of insulin: a feeding with medium or high carbohydrate intake.

The results of this study seem to indicate that the composition of the diet is able to influence overall energy expenditure, at least in some subjects. A subject very dear to Ludwig, who has been working for years to show that a diet rich in simple sugars favors the accumulation of fat, in open contrast with the official opinion that instead indicates the total caloric intake as a fundamental factor in weight control .

The study is very interesting and well conducted, variables and data distortion factors have been carefully checked and the measurement protocols used are the state of the art: however it is a single work that obviously needs further study, precisely because the results they go against what is shown by most of the studies available on the subject.

The reduction of carbohydrate intake could be indicated above all in a particular subgroup, that of those already based on high insulin levels, while the effect on the general population seems less relevant.

The authors point out that a similar effect could be obtained with controlled calorie intake and with a simultaneous reduction of the overall glycemic load, ie with the reduction of consumption of foods rich in simple sugars, those that are often referred to as junk foods. The authors are from the USA and this obviously affects their point of view: foods rich in sugars, drinks and snacks are consumed in significant quantities and in these conditions the simple transition to a richer diet of wholegrain products and vegetables can already be done wonders. In this sense, the study does not say anything particularly revolutionary but instead goes to confirm what has been gained by an impressive amount of previous work.

A low-carb diet - which is not necessarily a ketogenic diet or a paleo diet - can really be useful in a transition phase in those subjects who have high insulin secretion, a common situation among diabetic and obese individuals: if new jobs confirm the increase in energy expenditure linked to the composition of the diet detected by this study, it would be possible to draw up appropriate indications in the treatment of important and widespread diseases, obesity and diabetes first and foremost, more and more widespread diseases that have, among other things, an impact not negligible on public health costs.

For healthy subjects the best solution remains a varied diet, rich in vegetables, whole products, legumes and fruit - all foods with a modest glycemic load - far from any excess, with an adequate caloric intake compared to total energy expenditure. At this point the amount of carbohydrates present will be only a minor detail, like the handful of extra calories that the low-carb diet should allow to spend. It is better to work on your habits than to count on effects that, even if significant, are ultimately marginal compared to the overall picture of our lifestyle, so to be treated with every care.

Chapter 14: 15 Paleo recipes

Now it is the time to finish the book by taking a look at 15 of the best paleo recipes.

1. Ketogenic Pancakes

Ingredients:
1. 10 gr of butter
2. 3 eggs
3. 50 gr of sugar
4. 100 gr of milk
5. 200 gr of flour
6. jam
7. 1 package of baking powder
8. Nutella or jam

Preparation
1. Melt the butter and let it cool.
2. Divide the yolks from the whites.
3. Beat the egg whites until stiff and gradually add the sugar.
4. Beat the egg yolks with a whisk, adding the milk and butter.
5. Mix the flour together with the baking powder, sieve everything, and mix it a little at a time with the mixture of egg yolks, butter, and milk.
6. When the flour is finished, add the beaten egg whites until stiff and mix gently to avoid disassembling everything.
7. Use the mixture immediately so that it does not lose its softness.
8. Heat a nonstick plate together with a knob of butter. Pass it lightly with a sheet of kitchen paper to absorb excess butter.
9. Keeping the heat of the pan not too high, pour 1 ladle at a time of freshly prepared mixture.

10. As soon as bubbles appear on the surface, turn the pancakes with a fork. As they are ready, place them on top of each other on a plate and keep them warm.

Pancakes can be spread with Nutella or jam, but traditionally, they are eaten hot with plenty of Canadian maple syrup.

2. Ketogenic Meatballs

Ingredients for 4 servings
- 500 g of ground beef
- 1 whole egg
- 20 g of Parmesan cheese
- 20 g of breadcrumbs
- 1 clove of garlic
- 1/2 glass of white wine
- 100 g of carrots
- 1 tablespoon of fennel seeds
- 1 tablespoon of dried parsley
- Salt to taste
- 3 tablespoons of extra virgin olive oil

Preparation
- Let the lean butcher grind your lean meat, then season it with salt, the clove of garlic cut into small pieces, breadcrumbs, grated cheese, beaten egg and herbs.
- Mix everything well with your hands and if necessary adjust the consistency of the dough with the breadcrumbs if it is still not very compact. Shape the meatballs the size of a walnut.
- Wash, clean and slice the carrots on wheels, then heat the oil in a sufficiently large skillet and sauté the carrots and the meatballs over high heat, blending with white wine.
- Let evaporate for a few minutes, stirring well, stirring the pan by the handle (to avoid breaking the meatballs).

- Cover and cook over low heat for about 15-20 minutes, stirring occasionally to cook the meatballs on all sides. Serve the meatballs hot.

3. Spicy scrambled eggs

Ingredients for 2 servings
- 4 medium eggs
- 50 g of tuna in oil
- 1 teaspoon of mustard
- a pinch of pepper
- a pinch of salt
- chives and oregano
- 2 teaspoons of extra virgin olive oil
- 10 gr of mustard
- aromatic herbs (the ones you like the most)

Preparation
1. Place the eggs in a saucepan with water until covering and boiling for 15 minutes.
2. Allow the eggs to cool and peel them.
3. Cut them in half, take 3 egg yolks out of 4 and place them in a small bowl. Drain the tuna well from the preservation oil.
4. Mash the yolks with the tuna with a fork, add the mustard, pepper, salt and aromatic herbs. Once you have a smooth mixture, fill the egg whites.
5. Serve and season the eggs with oil and a sprinkling of pepper and herbs.
6. If you do not like the taste of mustard, you can replace it with curry powder or turmeric.

4. Ketogenic Biscuits

Ingredients for 10 servings
- *80 g chickpea flour*

- *90 g coconut flour (from pulp)*
- *30 ml extra virgin olive oil*
- *1 whole egg*
- *1 tablespoon of honey*
- *50 ml of coconut milk*
- *lemon peels*
- *1 pinch of salt*
- *2 teaspoons of ginger*
- *1 sachet of baking powder*

Preparation
1. Put the coconut flour, the chickpea flour, the pinch of salt, the ginger powder and the sachet of yeast in a bowl; mix well with a wooden spoon.
2. Grate the peel of an untreated lemon and add it to the flour.
3. Beat the egg with a whisk and add the honey first, then the oil and finally the milk, continuing to whisk with a whisk.
4. Combine the liquid ingredients with the flour and knead it well until you get a smooth ball. Remarry for half an hour.
5. Obtain 2-3 cm diameter balls from the dough and lay them in an oven-lined lacquer. Crush them with your hands to get the shape of biscuits.
6. Bake for 20-30 minutes at 170 ° C.

5. Vegetable passion

Ingredients
- 10 gr of butter
- 45 gr of pumpkin
- a table spoon of oil
- curry
- a pinch of salt
- a pinch of pepper
- 1 egg
- a pinch of walnut nutmeg

- 50 gr of parmesan

Preparation

1. You will need a small round baking dish (they are called ramekin); choose it high enough so that butter does not come out during the cooking process. To mix the ingredients, a small bowl is required and can be useful.
2. If you want to prepare several flans together to freeze them, you have to multiply them all the ingredients and the dishes; in any case, you will have to weigh all the items separately ingredients for each single flan (for 3 flans, 3 times 45 grams of pumpkin and not 135 grams of pumpkin).
3. Weigh separately all the ingredients; for the egg, mix thoroughly the yolk and light it with a whisk or a blender. Use a pumpkin that does not have too much water in it, such as Hokkaido (small, crushed, with dark green peel) or, better still, butternut (small with elongated neck).
4. Heat the oven to 180 degrees; cut the pumpkin into strips not too thin, put it on one pan with oven paper underneath; spray it with a spray (this oil is not weighed, with the spray will still be much less than one gram); spray over the curry (also unweighted, not exaggerated), salt and bake for 5 minutes in the ventilated oven.
5. Grease the ramekin (the bottom and the sides) well, with all the butter in the recipe; in bowl, stir egg, cream and almond flour; add a pinch of walnut nutmeg. Pull out the pumpkin and let it cool for two minutes. Pour the mixture into the ramekin and add the pumpkin.
6. At this point cover everything with grated Parmesan, spreading it in a uniformed manner (help yourself with a spatula). Bake for 25/30 minutes in the oven at 180 ° (ventilated); baked until there is one beautiful crust on the surface; it's not like a soufflé, so when you get it out of the oven it will not deflate. Served directly in the ramekin, it will remain warmer.

6. Keto Curry

Ingredients
- 10 gr of butter
- a tablespoon of olive oil
- 2 onions
- 1 package of curry
- 2 thyme leaves
- parsley
- fresh vegetables of your choice
- 100 gr of chicken
- 100 gr of rice

Preparation
1. To make the curry veal stew, heat the butter with oil in a pan and brown the chopped onions. When they have become transparent add the pieces of floured meat and brown them well over high heat turning them often because they take color evenly. After about five minutes add salt and pepper. In the meantime, melt the curry powder in a large glass of hot water.
2. Pour over the meat the curry dissolved in water, mix very well and cook covered, over medium-low heat for about an hour. Stir occasionally, and if the meat should dry out too much, add a little hot water.
3. When cooked, add the thyme leaves and the minced parsley. Transfer to the serving dish and serve the curry veal stew accompanied with pilaf rice or plain boiled rice.

7. Ketogenic Pasta

Ingredients
- 150 gr of spaghetti
- 1 lemon
- 10 gr of butter
- a pinch of salt

- 100 gr of ricotta

Preparation
1. To prepare spaghetti with lemon, place a pot with plenty of slightly salted water on the stove; as soon as it boils, cook the spaghetti according to the package directions.
2. In a pan melt the butter, add the lemon and stir for two minutes, then add the juice.
3. In a separate pan, toast the pine nuts taking care that they do not burn, then wash and dry the basil.
4. Drain the pasta keeping a glass of cooking water, add it to the lemon juice and mix well until it is all blended.
5. Add the Ricotta and a ladle of cooking water and mix well until it has formed a velvety cream that wraps the spaghetti.

8. Eggs and Tuna

Ingredients for 2 servings
- 4 medium eggs
- 50 g of tuna in oil
- 1 teaspoon of mustard
- a pinch of pepper
- a pinch of salt
- chives and oregano as you like
- 2 teaspoons of extra virgin olive oil
- other aromatic herbs (the ones you like)

Preparation
1. Place the eggs in a saucepan with water until covering and boiling for 15 minutes.
2. Allow the eggs to cool and peel them. Cut them in half, take 3 egg yolks out of 4 and place them in a small bowl. Drain the tuna well from the preservation oil.

3. Mash the yolks with the tuna with a fork, add the mustard, pepper, salt and aromatic herbs. Once you have a smooth mixture, fill the egg whites.
4. Serve and season the eggs with oil and a sprinkling of pepper and herbs.
5. If you do not like the taste of mustard, you can replace it with curry powder or turmeric.

9. Autumn tastes

Ingredients
- 100 gr of pork chop
- 1 pumpkin
- 10 gr of butter
- a tablespoon of olive oil
- a pinch of pepper
- a pinch of salt
- a tablespoon of soy sauce
- 25 gr of the cheese you like the most
- 2 potatoes
- 2 onions
- mixed vegetables

Preparation
1. To prepare the pork chops with pumpkin cream and cheese, first prepare the vegetable pieces, which will be used to prepare the pumpkin cream.
2. Then, dedicate yourself to the pumpkin cream: cut the pumpkin into slices, remove the outer peel, remove the seeds, then reduce the pulp first to strips and then into cubes. Peel the potatoes and cut into cubes too. Then take the onion, clean it and chop it finely, transfer it to a pan with the oil and sauté over a gentle heat.

3. Once the onion has reached the browning state, add the pumpkin in the pan together with the potatoes. Slowly add a few ladles of vegetable stock to cover the vegetables.
4. Season with salt and pepper and cook over low heat for 25-30 minutes, adding some vegetable stock occasionally. Once the vegetables are cooked, turn off the heat and start blending them with an immersion mixer until a smooth and homogeneous cream is obtained. Add a sprinkling of nutmeg and cinnamon and mix together; at this point your pumpkin cream is ready, so put it aside.
5. Take the chops and beat them with the meat until they are about 1 cm thick, then chop the sage and rosemary and place them in a non-stick pan with a little oil.
6. Put the chops in the pan, season with salt and pepper and leave to brown on both sides, turning them from time to time with a pincer so that they cook on both sides.
7. Once cooked, remove them from the pot and keep them warm. In the same pot in which they cooked the chops pour the previously prepared pumpkin cream, add the soy sauce and mix well.
8. Add the chops, season with the pumpkin cream, then cut the cheese into slices and place one above each chop. Cook for 1-2 minutes to melt the cheese, sprinkle everything with thyme leaves, mix well and your pork chops with pumpkin cream and cheese are ready to be served!

10. Taste of the sea

Ingredients
- 1 monkfish fillet
- pink pepper
- a pinch of salt
- a tablespoon of olive oil
- 200 gr of puff pastry
- 1 lemon

- 1 package of saffron
- mixed vegetables

Preparation
1. To prepare the monkfish in saffron and lemon sauce started with the cleaning of the monkfish fillet: cut into slices; with a knife remove the bones inside and then remove the skin. Cut the clean slices in half and make some tiny parts, tying them all around with the kitchen string: you need to prepare 8 monkfish medallions.
2. Remove the leaves from the thyme sprigs and place them on each nibble, then put the fish aside. Now take care of the sauce: in a pan pour oil, lemon; add the saffron bag and let it melt.
3. Add the pink pepper and thicken the sauce as well. Then sift the rice flour into the pan and mix well with a whisk to thicken the flour without creating lumps. Continuing with the whisk, pour the vegetable pieces as well; season it with salt and pepper and cook for a few minutes until the sauce becomes creamy.
4. Once ready, turn off the heat and set it aside. In another pan heat the oil and add the garlic. Once golden, remove the garlic and place the monkfish medallions.
5. Cook for a few minutes at medium heat and gently turn the tidbits with a kitchen tongs; when they have taken a nice brown color on both sides, turn off the heat. On a serving dish pour the saffron and lemon sauce (which will be the base on which to lay the fish) and place the monkfish medallions on it. Finish by pouring a few drops of sauce on the portions obtained and served.

11. Chicken and avocado

Ingredients
- 1 avocado

- ½ lemon
- 60 gr of oil
- salt
- parsley
- 100 gr of chicken
- 1 ginger

Preparation
1. For the recipe of chicken and avocado salad with ginger sauce, fry the chicken meat and pick it up in a bowl.
2. Peel the ginger and grate it, then squeeze the pulp in your hands, and pour the juice into a small bowl; add the juice of 1/2 lemon, 60 grams of oil, a pinch of salt, and parsley and blend with a dipping mixer to obtain a sauce.
3. Clean the avocado and cut into chunks. Season the chicken with the ginger sauce and complete with avocado chunks.
4. To make it taste better, you can also add the peeled lemon.

12. Cocoa and mint – a keto dessert

Ingredients
- 100 gr of butter
- 50 gr of coconut
- coconut oil
- peppermint extract
- cocoa powder

Preparation
1. Combine 100 of melted coconut butter, 50 grams of grated coconut, 1 tablespoon of coconut oil and half a teaspoon of peppermint extract.
2. Mix well and pour into cream puffs or muffin molds, filling them halfway.

3. Put in the fridge to harden (about 15 minutes).
4. Mix 2 tablespoons of melted coconut oil 2 tablespoons of cocoa powder.
5. Remove the peppermint mixture from the refrigerator and pour the cocoa mixture into each mold over the peppermint.
6. Refrigerate until the bombs harden.
7. Before serving, remove the bombs from the refrigerator and let them rest for about 5 minutes.

13. Rice and vegetables

Ingredients for 4 people
- 300 gr parboiled rice
- 160 gr tuna in drained oil
- 200 gr mozzarella cherries
- 120 gr pitted black olives
- 80 gr pesto
- extra virgin olive oil
- a pinch of salt
- 2 fresh basil leafs

Preparation

1) Boil in salted water 280 gr of parboiled rice, drained, seasoned with 80 gr of pesto and a little extra virgin olive oil, mix well and let it cool.
2) Add 120 gr black pitted olives, 200 g of cherry-cut mozzarella cut in half and finally 160 g of drained tuna and crumbled.
3) Sprinkle with a ground of pepper and mix well to flavor the rice.
4) Place the rice salad in the dishes, garnish it with some basil leaves and serve. If you want a more elegant presentation, grease a ring mold, pour the seasoned rice, crush a little

surface to fill all the holes well, and before serving, let stand for at least 10 minutes.
5) Turn the mold onto a serving dish, remove the mold and decorate with the basil leaves.

14. Ketogenic brioche

Ingredients
- 10 gr of butter
- 100 gr of flour
- 1 package of backing powder
- 50 gr of milk
- a pinch of sugar
- a pinch of salt

Preparation
1. Melt the butter and let it cool. Pour the flour into a bowl, add the baking powder, sugar and salt.
2. Stir, then incorporate the eggs, the melted butter and finally the milk.
3. Stir quickly with a fork, cover with the food foil and leave to rise for 3 hours at room temperature, in a warm place and away from drafts.
4. After this time, transfer the dough in the refrigerator and let it rest for 24 hours.
5. Before baking the brioche, leave it at room temperature for a couple of hours. Turn on the oven at 180 ° C, transfer the dough into a 23 cm long plum cake mold, with butter and flour.
6. Brush the surface with milk and decorate with the granulated sugar. Cook in the hot oven for about 40 minutes.

15. Ricotta explosion

Ingredients
- 150 gr of pasta
- 50 gr of ricotta
- Parmesan 30 gr
- a tablespoon of oil
- a pinch of salt
- a pinch of pepper

Preparation
1. To prepare this recipe, called "pasta and ricotta", first boil a pot of salt water and cook the pasta for 10 minutes or the time reported on the package.
2. In the meantime, you can prepare the dressing: using a spatula, sieve the ricotta in a bowl through a strainer with a tight mesh to obtain a nice smooth consistency.
3. Then add the grated Parmesan and fresh cream and mix well with the spatula. Add the thyme leaves, stir again, and finally add salt and pepper.
4. Drain the pasta, keeping some of its cooking water, and pour it directly into the bowl with the ricotta mixture;
5. mix well the pasta with the sauce, lengthening it with a ladle of cooking water, if necessary: your creamy pasta and ricotta is ready to be served!

1. Chocolate Chip Coconut Flour Cookies

Ingredients
1/3 cup + 2 Tbsp coconut flour
1/2 tsp baking soda
1/4 tsp sea salt
1/2 cup coconut oil, melted
1/2 cup coconut sugar
1/3 cup unsweetened coconut milk
3 eggs

1 tsp vanilla
2/3 cup chocolate chips (I recommend the "Enjoy Life" brand)

Instructions
Preheat the oven to 350F.

In a medium bowl, combine the coconut sugar & wet ingredients (coconut oil, coconut milk, eggs, & vanilla).

Add the remaining dry ingredients & chocolate chips, and stir until fully mixed.

Scoop the cookie dough onto a baking sheet lined with parchment paper. I used a cookie scoop.

You can use the bottom of a measuring cup to flatten the tops a bit if you want thinner cookies, just keep in mind that they will spread while baking.

Bake for 12-14 minutes, or until slightly firm to the touch.

2. Perfect Paleo Chocolate Chip Cookies

Ingredients
1 cup (100 grams) blanched almond flour
1/4 cup (32 grams) coconut flour
1 teaspoon baking soda
1/4 teaspoon salt
6 tablespoons (84 grams) coconut oil or unsalted butter, room temperature
3/4 cup (150 grams) coconut sugar or brown sugar
6 tablespoons (98 grams) natural almond butter, room temperature

1 1/2 teaspoons vanilla extract
1 large egg, room temperature
1 1/4 cups (213 grams) semi-sweet chocolate chips, divided

Instructions

In a medium mixing bowl, stir together the almond flour, coconut flour, baking soda and salt. Set aside.

In a large mixing bowl with an electric hand mixer or using a stand mixer, beat together the fat and sugar at medium speed until well combined, about 1 minute. If you use coconut oil, it may not come together easily. If that's the case, use your hands to combine it and then beat another 20 seconds.

Beat in the almond butter and vanilla extract on medium speed and mix until combined. Beat in the egg on low and mix until well incorporated. Stir in the flour mixture until well combined. Then stir in 1 cup (170 grams) chocolate chips. If you used brown sugar, skip to the next step. If you used coconut sugar, place the bowl in the refrigerator for about 1 hour or until the dough is firm.

Preheat the oven to 350 °F (175 °C) and line a baking sheet with a piece of parchment paper.

Roll the dough into 8 (75-gram) balls and place the remaining 1/4 cup (43 grams) of chocolate chips on the top and on the sides of the dough balls. You can also roll them into smaller balls but then you need to adjust the baking time. Place 3" apart on the prepared baking sheet. Press the cookies down lightly with the palm of your hand.

Bake for 11-14 minutes (if using coconut sugar) or 14-17 minutes (if using brown sugar) or until the surface of the center of the cookies no longer appears wet. They'll be very soft but will continue to cook as they sit on the cookie sheet.

Let cool completely on the baking sheet. Store in an airtight container for up to 3 days.

3. Crock Pot Paleo Cookies With Chocolate Chips

Ingredients
1/4 Cup Coconut oil, melted
1 Cup Coconut sugar
1 Large egg white
1/2 tsp Vanilla extract
1 1/2 Cups Finely ground almond meal (5.4oz)
1 3/4 tsp Baking powder
1/2 tsp Salt
1/2 Cup Dark chocolate chips

Instructions
Line a 5 quart crock pot with parchment paper and rub with coconut oil. Set aside.

In a large bowl, beat together the melted coconut oil and coconut sugar. Add in the egg white and vanilla extract and beat until well combined.

Pour the almond meal, baking powder and salt into the oil mixture and stir until well combined.

Stir in the chocolate chips.

Transfer the dough into the Crock pot and press down evenly. It can be a little tricky with the parchment paper.

Cook on LOW heat until the outside of the cookies appear golden brown, and the inside is still soft. About 2 - 2.5 hours. Be careful not to overcook the bars as they firm up A LOT once cooled.

Once cooked, carefully use the parchment paper as a handle and gently lift the bars out of the Crock pot* and transfer to a rack to cool completely.

Once cooled, cut and devour.

4. Farmer Boys Delight Paleo Cookie

Ingredients
1/2 cup coconut oil, room temperature
3/4 cup coconut sugar
1 egg, room temperature
1 teaspoon vanilla extract
1/2 teaspoon baking soda
1/2 teaspoon salt
2 1/4 cups (9 oz.) almond flour (I recommend Honeyville blanched almond flour)
1 cup (6 oz.) chopped dark chocolate

Directions
Preheat the oven to 350ºF.

Beat together the coconut oil and coconut sugar until smooth. Add the egg and vanilla and mix until smooth.

Add the almond flour, salt, and baking soda to the wet ingredients. Mix until well incorporated.

Fold in the chopped chocolate. Cover with plastic wrap and refrigerate for at least an hour (can prepare up to 48 hours ahead of time).

After refrigerating, use a cookie scoop to form cookies and press down slightly. Bake for 10 minutes or just beginning to turn golden brown around the edges.

5. Chewy Grain Free Snickerdoodles

Ingredients
1/2 cup butter or coconut oil, softened
1/2 cup coconut sugar
1/4 cup pure maple syrup
1 large egg
1 tsp pure vanilla extract
2 cups blanched almond flour
1/2 tsp baking soda
1/4 tsp cream of tartar
1/4 tsp salt

For rolling in
1/4 cup coconut sugar
2 tsp cinnamon

Instructions
Using a standmixer fitted with the paddle attachment, beat together the butter or coconut oil, coconut sugar, and syrup on medium-high speed until well combined and creamy.

Scrape down sides and add in egg and vanilla and beat together again until creamy.

Sift in the almond flour, baking soda, cream of tartar and salt. Beat until combined.

Scoop out with a cookie scoop onto a baking sheet covered with parchment paper.

Place in fridge for about an hour, until chilled.

Preheat oven to 350 degrees.

Flatten slightly and roll in the cinnamon/coconut sugar mixture until covered.

Bake in oven for 8-9 minutes, then remove from oven and allow to cool on baking sheet for 4-5 minutes before removing to wire rack to cool completely.

Note: It's important this dough is chilled when you place it in the oven. This will help ensure a bit of a crispy outside, and soft, chewy center.

6. Carrot Cake Caveman Cookies

Ingredients
2 cups mini carrots
2 cups almonds
1 cup shredded coconut
1 tsp nutmeg
2 tsp vanilla
2 tsp coconut oil
3 eggs

Instructions
Preheat your oven to 350 Degrees F.

Combine all of your ingredients EXCEPT your eggs in a food processor, pulse it until all the pieces are small but still a little chunky.

Combine that mixture with the eggs in a large mixing bowl and mix well.

Using your hands, form the mixture into "patties" and place on a parchment paper lined cookie sheet. The size of the "patties" are up to you, or you could make the into bars.

Bake until done, around 35-40 Minutes.

7. Avocado Banana Cookies

Ingredients
1 cup very ripe avocado flesh
1 banana
1 egg
1/2 cup dark cocoa powder
2 tbsp. raw honey (optional)
Dark chocolate chunks, to taste
1/2 tsp. baking soda

Instructions
Preheat your oven to 350 F.

Combine the banana, avocado, and honey in a bowl.

Mix everything until smooth using a hand mixer or a food processor.

Add in the egg, baking soda, and cocoa powder, and continue mixing until everything is well blended.

Stir in the dark chocolate chunks, if using.

Drop spoonfuls of cookie dough on a baking sheet lined with parchment paper. The dough will be very soft.

Bake for 8 to 10 minutes or until the cookies are warm and firm.

8. Huge Paleo Cookie for one Person

Ingredients
3 T coconut flour, sifted
1 T almond flour (can sub for an extra T coconut flour)
2 T granulated sweetener of choice
pinch cinnamon
pinch sea salt
1 scoop protein powder of choice (optional)
2 T nut butter of choice (I used crunchy almond butter)
1 T pure maple syrup (can sub for any sweetener of choice)
1-2 T mix ins of choice (I used cashews, dairy free chips and almonds)
1/4 cup Silk Unsweetened Vanilla Almond milk

Instructions
In a large mixing bowl, combine the flours, sweetener of choice, cinnamon, sea salt and protein powder if using it. Mix well.

Add in the nut butter of choice and maple syrup and mix until a thick, crumbly mixture remains.

Add your mix ins of choice. Using a tablespoon at a time, at your your Silk Almond Milk until a very thick batter is formed.

Using your hands, form into a large ball and press firmly onto a lined plate. Eat as it is or refrigerate for 20-30 minutes for a firm cookie.

9. Soft & Chewy Double Chocolate Cookies

Ingredients
1 cup thick almond butter (I used Barney Butter Smooth Almond Butter because it's similar to thick nut butters. If you use too oily, the cookies won't come together. You were warned.)
1 cup coconut sugar
1 egg, whisked
1/2 cup unsweetened cocoa powder
1 teaspoon baking soda
1 teaspoon vanilla extract
pinch of salt
1/4-1/2 cup Enjoy Life Mini Chocolate Chips

Instructions
Preheat oven to 350 degrees.

In a large bowl, mix together almond butter and coconut sugar using a large spoon. Then add egg and mix again until well combined.

Add 1/4 cup of cocoa powder at a time. At this point, I used my hands to incorporate the cocoa powder into the dough. Add all the cocoa powder and completely combine.

Then add baking soda, vanilla, salt and chocolate chips and combined until everything is well mixed. This was all hands for me. It's a dirty job, but someone has to do it. (This should be a very thick dough at this point. If it's not, you need a thicker almond butter like I said before).

Use a cookie scoop to scoop out around 2 tablespoons of dough and make into a round ball. Place on silpat or parchment paper lined baking sheet. This dough will create 13-15 cookies that size.

Once you've placed all the balled dough onto the baking sheet, use a fork to press the cookies down just slightly. No need to really flatten them out, just get them to look more cookie shape instead of ball shape. If you press them down too much, they'll come apart when they bake so be careful.

Place baking sheet into the oven and bake for 10 minutes.

Remove from oven and let cool for 5-10 minutes until removing from baking sheet to place on cooling rack. If you try to remove these from the baking sheet early, they will come apart. So don't be stupid here. Patience is a virtue. Eat up!

10. Paleo Hazelnut Cookies

Ingredients
100 grams blanched hazelnut flour
150 grams blanched almond flour (about 1-1/2 cups)
1/4 teaspoon baking soda
1/8 teaspoon sea salt
1/4 cup melted grass-fed organic ghee
1/4 cup honey
1 teaspoon vanilla extract

Instructions
Preheat oven to 325 degrees.

Combine dry ingredients in large bowl. Combine wet ingredients in small. Pour wet ingredients into dry, and stir until a thick dough is formed.

Use a small cookie scoop, scoop onto baking sheet lined with parchment paper. Use a small piece of parchment to flatten cookies to 1/4 inch thick.

Bake until just starting to brown, 10-12 minutes. Cool on wire rack.

11. Paleo Pumpkin Spice Chocolate Chip Cookies

Ingredients
1 1/2 cup almond flour, blanched
1/2 cup pumpkin puree, organic
3 tablespoon almond butter
1/4 cup honey, raw
1/4 cup coconut oil, melted
2 teaspoon vanilla
1 teaspoon baking soda
1 tablespoon pumpkin pie spice
1/2 cup chocolate chips, semi-sweet, Enjoy Life Mini Chips

Instructions
Preheat oven to 350 F.

Line a baking sheet with parchment paper.

In a small mixing bowl, combine dry ingredients (almond flour, baking soda, pumpkin pie spice).

Set aside.

In a food processor (or a medium bowl with a hand mixer), beat together the wet ingredients (pumpkin puree, almond butter, honey, melted coconut oil, vanilla extract).

Mix dry ingredients into the wet ingredients until well combined. Stir in chocolate chips.

Drop tablespoon size balls of cookie dough onto the prepared baking sheet. Press them down to flatten (if desired).

Bake approximately 10-12 minutes or until the tops are golden brown.

Remove baking sheet from oven, and let cookies sit for a few moments to cool. They will be slightly soft, but they will harden as they cool.

After 5 minutes, move cookies to a wire rack to finish cooling.

Enjoy! For a crispier cookie, put them into the freezer and enjoy cold.

12. Probably The Healthiest Cookies in the World.

Ingredients
1 1/2 cups raw walnut halves
1 cup medjool dates, pitted (about 12)
1/4 teaspoon salt
1/2 teaspoon baking soda
1 teaspoon vanilla extract

1 flax egg (1 tablespoon ground flax or chia seeds + 3 tablespoons water)
1/2 cup dark chocolate chips (optional)

Instructions
Preheat the oven to 350F and line a baking sheet with parchment paper or a silpat.

In the bowl of a food processor fitted with an "S" blade, process the dates and walnuts together until a crumbly texture is formed. Add in the salt, baking soda, vanilla and flax egg and process again until the batter is relatively smooth. Add in the chocolate chips and briefly pulse, just to combine.

Spoon the batter onto a lined baking sheet, and use your hands to gently flatten the cookie dough. (Tip: Wet your hands with water to prevent sticking!) Bake at 350F for 12 minutes, or until the edges are slightly golden. Allow to cool on the pan for 10 minutes, then transfer the cookies to a wire rack to cool completely.

Serve immediately, and store the leftovers in a sealed container in the fridge or freezer for best shelf life. These cookies should last a week in the fridge, and a month or more in the freezer.

13. Paleo Toffee Bar Recipe

Ingredients
2 cups unsweetened shredded coconut
1/2 cup coconut sugar
1/3 cup coconut oil, melted
2 eggs
1 teaspoon vanilla extract
1/2 teaspoon salt

1 cup dairy free chocolate chips

Instructions
Preheat oven to 350 degrees F.

Line a 9X13 inch baking dish with parchment paper.

Mix together coconut, coconut sugar, coconut oil, eggs, vanilla and salt.

Press into baking dish evenly.

Bake for 25-30 minutes, until set and lightly browned.

Turn off oven, remove pan and sprinkle with chocolate chips. Return to oven for a few minutes so that chocolate chips can melt, then spread melted chips with a butter knife or offset spatula.

Allow to cool so chocolate can re-harden.

Cut into squares. Serve immediately or store in freezer.

14. Flourless Mexican Hot Chocolate Brownie Cookies

Ingredients
3 cups of Powdered Coconut Sugar
1 cup Dutch Processed Cocoa
1/2 teaspoon Salt
1 tablespoon Ground Cinnamon
1 and 1/2 teaspoon McCormick Cocoa Chili Powder
3 or 4 egg-whites
1 teaspoon Vanilla

1 cup Semi-Sweet Chocolate Chips (Enjoy Life Brand is paleo friendly)

Instructions

Preheat the oven to 320 degrees and put your oven's two baking racks in the bottom third and top third of your oven.

Put the powdered coconut sugar, cocoa, salt, cinnamon, and cocoa-chili powder into the bowl of a stand-mixer. Whisk till throughouly combined. (depending on the depth of your bowl and whisk attachment, you may need to scrape the sides and/or scrap the bottom with a spatula to ensure the dry ingredients are completely mixed).

Add 3 egg-whites and the one teaspoon of vanilla, whisking to combine. The batter should be in a very thick brownie-batter like state. If it is too dry, add the 4th egg white. Fold in the semi-sweet chocolate chips.

Using a 1-tablespoon cookie scoop, scoop batter onto two parchment lined cookie sheets, leaving 1 inch in between each cookie.

Place both cookie sheets in the preheated oven and bake 8 minutes. Rotate the pans between the top and bottom racks and bake another 9-10 minutes.

Remove the pans from the oven and let cool one-two minutes. Test a cookie by attempting to remove it from the parchment; if it removes easily, the cookies have completely baked and you can move the parchment paper of cookies onto a wire rack to completely cool. IF the cookie sticks to the parchment when you attempt to remove it, return the cookie sheet to the oven and cook another 2-3 minutes.

Once completely cooled, store in an air-tight container.

15. Paleo Macadamia Cranberry Cookies

Ingredients
3/4 cup whole raw macadamia nuts
1/2 cup dried cranberries, roughly chopped
1 cup almond flour or almond meal
1 cup unsweetened fine desiccated coconut
1/2 tsp ground ginger
1/4 tsp to 1/2 tsp ground nutmeg (depending on your taste)
1/4 cup honey
1/4 cup coconut oil, melted
1/2 tsp baking soda
2 tbsp water, divided

Instructions
Preheat oven to 320F/160C. Line two baking sheets with parchment paper.

Arrange macadamia nuts on a baking sheet in a single layer and bake for 6 to 8 minutes or until lightly toasted. Let them cool and chop them roughly.

Reduce oven to 250F/120C.

In a large bowl, combine almond flour, desiccated coconut, macadamia, cranberries, ginger and nutmeg.

In a small saucepan, combine honey and coconut oil and melt gently over low heat. Mix baking soda with 1 tablespoon water and stir in honey/coconut oil mixture. Once the mixture froths up (this will only take a few seconds), remove from heat and pour on the dry ingredients. Add 1 tablespoon of water and mix well during 1-2 minutes.

Form balls with the batter using a medium cookie/ice cream scoop (or about 1 1/2 tablespoons).

Place them on the lined baking sheet and flatten them using the palm of your hand. They won't spread so shape them as neatly and roundly as you can. You should get about 14 cookies.

Bake for 30 minutes or until golden. Remove from the oven and leave to cool completely, as they will be too fragile to pick up when still warm.

16. Paleo Gingersnap Cookies

Ingredients
1/2 cup melted palm shortening (or grass fed butter)
1 cup coconut/palm sugar
1 egg
1 Tbs real maple syrup
1 tsp unsulfured blackstrap molasses
1 tsp pure vanilla extract
2 tsp fresh grated ginger
1 1/2 cup tapioca flour
3 Tbs coconut flour, divided
2 tsp baking soda
1/8 tsp fine grain sea salt
1 Tbs ground ginger
1 tsp cinnamon
1/4 tsp allspice
3 Tbs raw cane sugar for rolling the cookies (optional)

Instructions

Using an electric mixer with a whisk attachment. Beat together the melted palm shortening and coconut/palm sugar, scraping down the sides of the bowl with a spatula as needed.

Add the egg, maple syrup, molasses, vanilla extract, and fresh grated ginger. Mix until well incorporated.

In a separate bowl, whisk together the: tapioca flour, coconut flour, baking soda, sea salt, ground ginger, cinnamon, and allspice. Slowly sift the dry mixture into the wet ingredients, mixing on a low speed. Stop to scrape down the sides of the bowl with a spatula as needed.

Turn up the speed to medium and mix until well incorporated.

Transfer the dough to the refrigerator to set up for 30 minutes. I use this time to preheat my oven and clean up my kitchen.

Preheat oven to 325 degrees.

Scoop 1 rounded teaspoon of chilled dough, per cookie. Roll the dough into a ball 1" ball. If you want to add a little sparkle, you can roll the balls in a plate of organic cane sugar. This step is optional.
Place dough balls onto a baking sheet lined with parchment paper. Leave room for the cookies to spread, they will be approximately 2 & 1/2" wide. I suggest no more than nine cookies per sheet.

Bake for approximately 10 minutes in a 325-degree oven. Oven temperatures vary, so keep an eye on them. They should be golden brown and look crispy.

Allow cookies to cool before serving. Store extra cookies wrapped tightly in the freezer.

17. Flourless Cashew Butter Chocolate Chip Cookies

Ingredients
1/2 cup coconut sugar
1 large egg
1 cup cashew butter (or almond butter, or your favorite nut butter)
1 teaspoon baking soda
1 1/2 teaspoon vanilla extract
Pinch of salt
2/3 cup dairy-free mini chocolate chips

Instructions
Preheat oven to 350 degrees Fahrenheit and line baking sheets with parchment paper or silicone baking mats.

In a large bowl, whisk together coconut sugar and egg until incorporated. Add in the cashew butter, baking soda, vanilla extract, and salt. Mix with a spatula or wooden spoon until batter comes together. Stir in the chocolate chips.

Using a medium cookie scoop, scoop dough and roll into a ball then place on baking sheet.

Bake for 10 minutes and let cool on cookie sheet for 5 minutes before transferring them to a wire rack to cool completely.

Store in an airtight container for up to 1 week.

18. Skinny Chocolate Peanut Butter No Bake Cookies

Ingredients
1/2 cup (125g) creamy peanut butter (or crunchy; if using natural style peanut butter make sure it is not oily)
1 small very ripe banana, mashed (about 1/3 cup)
1/3 cup (113g) honey (or maple syrup or agave)
1/4 cup (22g) unsweetened cocoa powder
1/4 cup (60ml) milk (coy, almond, soy)
3 cups (240g) quick-cooking oats
1/8 teaspoon salt
1/3 cup (60g) mini chocolate chips, optional

Instructions
Line a baking sheet with parchment paper or a silicone baking mat. Set aside.

Melt peanut butter and mashed banana together in a large skillet over low heat until fully melted and combined. Remove from heat and mix in the honey, cocoa powder, milk, oats, and salt. The mixture will be thick and fudgy.

Drop cookie dough (about 2 Tablespoons per cookie) on the baking sheet, molding the cookie into desired shape. Press a few mini chocolate chips onto tops, if desired.

Place in the refrigerator for at least 2 hours before enjoying.

Makes 16 cookies. Cookies remain fresh up to 10 days stored (covered) in the refrigerator. Cookies freeze well up to 3 months.

19. Peppermint Chocolate Crinkle Cookies

Ingredients
2 1/2 cups almond meal
2 T coconut flour
2 T cocoa powder
1/2 cup coconut palm sugar + 1/4 cup ground coconut palm sugar for rolling*
1/2 tsp baking soda
1/2 tsp salt
2 large eggs
1/4 cup coconut oil, melted
1/4 cup dairy-free chocolate chips, melted (I use Enjoy Life brand)
1 tsp peppermint extract

Instructions
In a large bowl combine almond meal, coconut flour, cocoa powder, 1/2 cup coconut palm sugar, baking soda and salt.

In a separate bowl combine eggs, coconut oil, chocolate chips and pepper extract.

Add the wet ingredients to the dry and stir until just combined.

Cover bowl and place in fridge for one hour (or overnight) or freezer for 20 minutes. Dough should harden. Do not skip

Preheat oven to 350 degrees F.

Scoop out 1 tablespoon worth of dough and roll into a ball between palms.

Roll each ball in 1/4 cup of ground coconut palm sugar to coat.

Place balls on a parchment or silicone lined baking sheet and bake for 10 minutes.

Remove from oven and let sit on tray for 10 minutes before removing to cool completely on a wire rack. Do not try to remove before 10 minutes as they will be too soft.

Dust with any leftover ground coconut palm sugar for a more "snowball" like effect.

Will keep for several days in an airtight container on your countertop.

20. Orange Blossom Cookies

Ingredients
3 cups almond flour
1/4 cup coconut flour
1/3 cup coconut oil, melted
Zest of 1 large navel orange
1 Tbsp organic vanilla extract
1/2 tsp aluminum-free baking soda
pinch unrefined sea salt
1/3 cup honey (preferably local raw)
1/3 cup fresh orange juice (from 1/2 navel orange)

Instructions
Preheat oven to 350 F

Place all ingredients in a glass bowl and blend well with a pastry blender

Form a large ball with the dough and place on wax paper. Put this in the freezer for 15 minutes (the cookies will stay together better this way)

Form 1-1.5 inch balls with the dough and place on a cookie sheet

Press dough balls down with a wet fork creating a cross hatch pattern. Wet the fork after every cookie to prevent the dough from sticking

Bake for 13-15 minutes (until tops are golden brown)

Remove from oven, let cool, and enjoy!

21. Maple Bacon Chocolate Chip Cookies

Ingredients
4 Slices of Bacon
2-3 Tbsp. Bacon Fat
1 Cup Almond Flour
1/2 Cup Chocolate Chips {I like Enjoy Life Chocolate Chips}
2 Eggs
3 Tbsp. Maple Syrup {Get the good stuff!}
1 tsp. Vanilla Extract

Instructions
Preheat your oven to 350{F}

Cook your bacon in a pan and save the fat! It's highly suggested that you make yourself an extra few slices to munch on.

While it's cooking I like to combine all my other ingredients {except for the bacon and bacon fat} and mix well.

When the bacon is done, chop it up into 1/4-1/2" pieces, we like the pieces bigger around here because it gives better flavor / texture.

When you add the bacon into the bowl make sure you break it up with your fingers so all the bacon doesn't stay in one spot. And add the bacon fat. Mix it all well!

On a baking sheet (I line mine w/ aluminum foil to save on clean up) use a teaspoon measure and do heaping scoops and if needed pat them out to be a little bit flatter/ more even.

Bake for 8-10 minutes, until the edges are a little golden and the center is firm to the touch.

If you can let them cool. If not just dive right in!

Conclusion

Thank you for making it to the end of this book, we really appreciate your interest in the paleo diet. Now you have got all the information you need to start changing your lifestyle and getting back in shape. It is always a pleasure to see our readers turn their health around after reading our books and we know you will be the next success story.

We would like to end this book by encouraging you to take the first step. We know, it is always the most difficult, but we also know that once you have done it, everything becomes easier. During the first days of the paleo diet, we suggest you to listen to your body more than ever: it will be amazing to see how it starts transforming, using the new patterns you are offering it.

This is your time, this is the moment when your health begins a new journey. Stay consistent, stay motivated.

You got this!

Part 2

Introduction

Food is a vital function that provides the essential nutritional elements for good physical, psychological and emotional health. Food is also a social, family and cultural practice that allows you to take a seat in your family and social environment (family meals, outings to restaurants, traditions and religious holidays).

In addition, nutrition plays a preventive role in the onset or development of certain diseases such as obesity, diabetes, high blood pressure or cardiovascular diseases, when it is too rich, too fat or too sweet. It is important to try to maintain a stable weight, which demonstrates a balanced diet. The 3 meals a day (morning, noon and night), allow the person to keep a rhythm of food and a balance of health in the long term, necessary to a healthy and harmonious state of mind.

The diet is individually adapted because the calorie needs vary according to the person, according to their age, their weight, their gender (female or male), their energy expenditure and their physical activity performed. In this book, you will have the opportunity to learn more on how to lose weight and get healthy eating the right food for your body +3 weeks' diet plan. Enjoy the reading!

Chapter One

Eating, Diet, and Nutrition to Healthy living

Nourishing your body is the most natural and essential action of your everyday life. Day after day, every meal involves making food choices, whether conscious or automatic. But do your choices help improve your health and quality of life?

In recent decades, nutrition-related rates of obesity and chronic diseases have increased, although we are becoming more informed about the benefits of good nutrition. There are several factors that can influence your decisions and your eating habits: foods in schools, groceries and restaurants, marketing and social exchanges, or simply lack of information on less nutritious foods. Collectively, the minds of the population, aging well, is knowing how to keep good health and maintain a physical form in spite of passing years. However, do you think the physical condition is enough to age well? We will see that to experience aging in a positive way it is important to maintain both one's body and one's mind in good health. For that, there are keys like to stay as long as possible active and autonomous and to take general measures concerning their way of life.

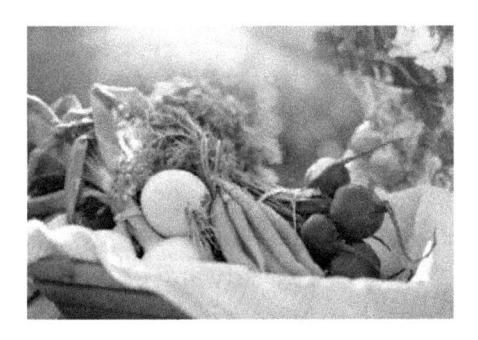

The body needs food to function well, for this reason, it is advisable to vary the food in reasonable quantity (eat fruits, vegetables, sugars, fats, legumes, dairy products, meat, eggs, fish, etc.) Water is also very important to the proper functioning of the body. Other drinks, such as coffee, tea, fruit juice, can also be drunk moderately. Also, some foods are known to be beneficial for intelligence, memory, and concentration (fish, all fruits and vegetables, or some food supplements such as wheat, oats, rye, sesame, etc.). On the other hand, it is better to avoid excessive consumption of saturated fats (charcuterie, whole dairy, cheese, butter) and red meats.

At any point in time of one's life, it is essential to engage in daily physical activity as it gives lasting positive health effects, improves quality of life, resistance to fatigue, contributes to the quality of sleep and improves physical fitness.

It should be noted that regular sports practice improves emotional well-being, physical well-being, quality of life (subjective well-being) and self-perception. Studies of the benefits of physical activity show that the risk of premature death is lower in physically active people than in others.

For the adults and the elderly, practicing sporting activities with gentle methods like gymnastics, yoga, walking, is appropriate for keeping muscles and joints in good condition.

However, good food hygiene and the practice of regular physical activity are the first means of prevention to preserve effectively its health capital and to maintain its quality of life and its autonomy.

Being good on your head also helps you feel better. Here are some tips for a healthy lifestyle, which may allow some to reduce the risk of health problems and live more harmoniously:

Have a good philosophy of life:
- Make yourself useful to society and others
- To question oneself to always evolve.
- Enjoy the good moments of life

- Maintain a varied intellectual life by watching the news, reading the newspaper, playing, traveling, staying curious and active
- Ability to stimulate your mind by making memory games, concentration such as Sudoku, Scrabble, arrow words, crosswords, and many others.
- **Cultivate your social life: meet new people, go out (go to the cinema, restaurant), be part of an association, etc.**

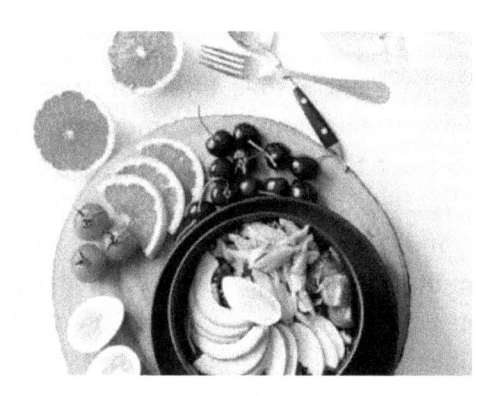

Although our eating habits have a direct impact on our health. A balanced diet is one of the essential components, if not the most essential component, of a healthy life. Many people do not pay much attention to their food choices because they do not realize how powerful food allies can be.

When you eat healthy foods, your body gets the nutrients it needs: vitamins, minerals and fiber, fiber, (healthy) fats, carbohydrates, protein, and these will strengthen the immune system, repair the damage of body, build new healthy cells, recover after an effort and fight against diseases.

The problem with our modern eating habits is that:
1. With our hectic lives, we often end up eating what is practical, rather than what is healthy.
2. Many common foods contain small amounts of nutrients.

3. Fast food, ready meals, and junk food are highly processed. Processing removes a lot of the nutrients, and these foods are often filled with unhealthy ingredients such as chemicals, preservatives, sodium, sugars, and artificial flavors.

Eating these unhealthy foods on a regular basis can cause undernourishment even if you eat a lot of food. And since these are calories without nutritional value, your body does have the nutrients it needs (even if you fill your stomach).

The best choice is to focus on healthy foods. Focus on good foods like fruits and vegetables, beans and legumes, nuts and seeds (whole grains).

The most immediate and visible effect of poor food hygiene on our health is weight gain, and sometimes even obesity. But this is the visible side of the iceberg because then come problems like diabetes, heart disease, high blood pressure, underweight, weak bones, and sometimes even depression or problems cognitive. A multitude of other problems and pathologies not listed here can occur in the medium-long term if you make the wrong food choices. Diet is the key to good health!

Eating well does not just mean eating soups, eating less, or saying no to fat. Healthy eating habits mean a nutritious diet, that is, eating everything in the right amount and in the right way. Do not completely exclude fat and do not overdo it with fiber and protein! Do not forget that you have to provide children with a good balance of all types of foods, because it is the age for physical and mental development. And finally, forget the processed foods, limit to the maximum sugar, salt, white flour, and some might tell you to limit also the cow's milk (the famous 4 whites).

BENEFITS OF A HEALTHY DIET

1. MAINTAIN ONE'S FITNESS WEIGHT

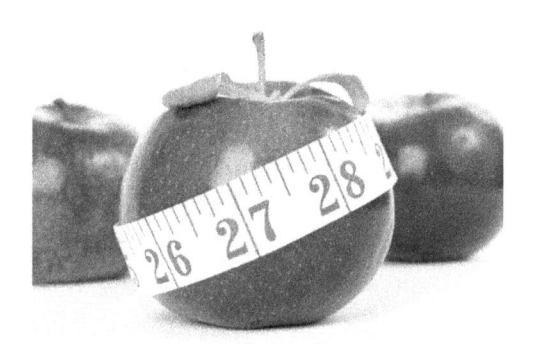

Exercising regularly and eating well can help you maintain a healthy weight and avoid getting fat. It is, therefore, preferable to maintain good food hygiene over time rather than trying to catch up with diets. When you stop dieting, you will almost always regain all the weight you have lost. All your efforts to lose weight will have been useless.

2. DISEASE CONTROL

By lowering unhealthy triglycerides and promoting good cholesterol, good dietary choices can prevent many dangerous health problems. Some foods are anti-oxidants and anti-inflammatories, which avoids the damage caused by free radicals. When a diet is healthy, it assists your body to minimize the risk of cardiovascular disease. Obesity, diabetes, cancer, high blood pressure, heart disease, stroke, and osteoporosis are all consequences of poor eating habits.

3. KEEP YOUR BRAIN IN GOOD SHAPE

A diet that is healthy is as good for your brain as it is for the rest of your body system. Unhealthy foods are linked to a whole series of neurological problems. Some nutritional deficiencies increase the risk of depression. Other nutrients, such as potassium, are involved in the functioning of brain cells. A varied and healthy diet keeps your brain functioning and can also promote good mental health.

4. DECREASE THE RISK OF CANCER

Fruits and vegetables are loaded with antioxidants, which are substances that seek out and neutralize potentially harmful cells (free radicals). Free radicals contain an unequal amount of electrons, which makes them very unstable. When they search for and steal electrons in healthy cells, they can cause damage. Antioxidants neutralize the body by freeing radicals and donating one of their electrons, turning the free radical into a stable molecule.

5. CONTROL OF BLOOD GLUCOSE

Sweet foods such as white bread, fruit juice, soft drinks, and ice cream cause a spike in blood sugar. Although your body can handle occasional surges of glucose, over time this can lead to insulin resistance, which can turn into type 2 diabetes. Complex carbohydrates, such as whole grain bread, oatmeal oats, and brown rice, cause a slow release of sugar in the blood, which helps to regulate blood sugar.

6. A LONGER LIFE AND QUALITY

To be healthy, in addition to a healthy diet, you should start exercising, quit smoking, start monitoring your cholesterol levels, your blood pressure, and your weight. Eating healthy is more a part of a lifestyle change than a diet. You will gradually feel the need to feel good about all aspects of your life.

Chapter Two

Why Paleo Diet?

A diet can be followed as a therapeutic or preventive treatment of a disease. Many people decide to diet to refine their silhouette and lose the famous "extra pounds." A diet is prescribed by a doctor to treat health problems therapeutically or preventively. Going on a diet helps to treat, relieve or reduce a patient's symptoms, such as diabetes, cardiovascular risks, overweight, and a food allergy.

Paleo is one of the healthiest ways to eat because it uses a nutritional approach that relies on genetics to keep your body slim, strong and enthusiastic. Research in most food and nutrition expertise and the Paleo review show that this diet is the modern full of refined foods.

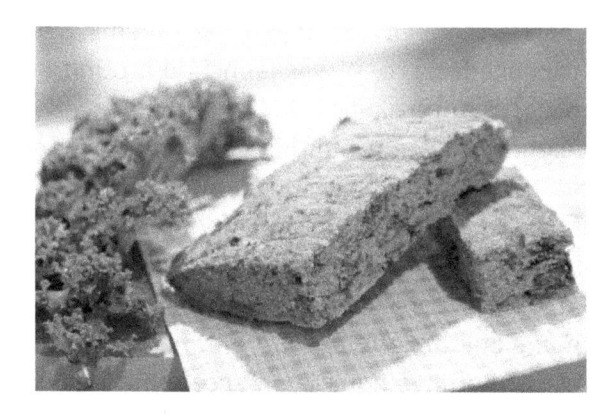

Paleo diet is also called the Caveman diet, Hunter-gatherer diet, Paleolithic diet or Stone Age diet. It's become popular among most lovers of. This usually includes eating what people in the Paleolithic eat, such as lean meats, fruits, vegetables, nuts, and seeds. However, a Paleo diet limits foods such as dairy products, legumes, and cereals.

What Is the Right Choice for You?
Although the Paleo diet is not the best for anyone who does not agree with some of its dietary limitations, it a proven fact that it provides a healthy alternative for those who desire to lose weight and improve their health. General like any other market, this diet must have a balance between all the foods eaten. This program allows you to get all the nutrients the body needs without eating too much. This diet is the perfect choice for you because it is a natural way to lose weight with less risk to your health.

The Paleolithic Diet, also known as the Caveman Diet, is a diet modeled on the eating habits of humans or rather our Homo habilis ancestor of the Paleolithic age that began about 2.5 millions of years. Although the Paleo diet seems new, it was revived several decades ago. It was launched around the 70s by the American gastroenterologist Walter Voegtlin with the idea that our ancestors of the Paleolithic could teach modern men how to eat healthily.

When we eat Paleo, we eliminate all foods containing salt or sugar, or dairy products, cereals, legumes, but also refined oils appeared for 10,000 years. Indeed, our DNA has remained the same since the Paleolithic era, but our diet has changed radically from that time, and things have even accelerated over the past 50 years. The food that we are adapted to, that which allows us to be the fittest and healthy, would be that of the Paleolithic: fresh food from hunting or gathering (meat, fish, poultry, eggs, vegetables and fruits, nuts and seeds, herbs and spices).

Paleo has been known for several years now, but it has never been so seduced. Unlike other diets, it was not "designed" by a nutritionist since it corresponds to what the first humans ate naturally. It is based on the assumption that modern food is not genetically adapted to our species and that we should eat like the first hominids who were "hunter-gatherers." In other words, our genetic heritage has not changed in 40,000 years while food models, they have completely changed, especially since the development of livestock and agriculture in the Neolithic.

It is this shift that gradually introduced degenerative diseases that our ancestors probably did not know. The researchers even think that they would be able to compete with the best modern athletes. Some, like Dr. Jean Seignalet, who died in 2003, have even used this diet against autoimmune diseases such as multiple sclerosis, rheumatoid arthritis or fibromyalgia, three diseases that traditional medicine is struggling to treat.

For several years now, researchers have been striving to identify precisely the composition of this prehistoric regime. Even if no consensus really emerges, researchers agree on different points: during the Paleolithic, dairy products, cereals (including bread) and legumes were not part of it. Salty foods, refined sugar, soft drinks, and processed foods either. On the other hand, it seems that the paleo diet was richer in protein and fat than the modern diet. But unlike the programs richly documented by some books. Beyond the lack of knowledge about the eating habits of our ancestors, the Paleolithic regime, so attractive, comes up against several limits.

As you can see, the paleo diet favors foods available in the Paleolithic era. It, therefore, focuses on quality in the foods you eat because they are fresh, whole, natural and these are the ones that contain more vitamins and minerals. It is the guarantee of better health, mood, recovery, performance and also less risk of injury and inflammation in general.

It is an excellent diet that will bring you many benefits and can be followed by any person (sports or not) wanting to lose fat and regain vitality while being satiated. You understand it; it's not just a "diet" but a way to eat which is synonymous with common sense.

Be aware, however, that we are able to digest certain modern foods (except cases of intolerance) that appeared later on the scale of human evolution. They should not be the basis of your diet but can benefit athletes whose physical activity requires a higher intake of carbohydrates and proteins or simply by the question of taste and desires. These are cereals (preferably gluten-free), legumes (making sure they are soaked), dairy products, preferably raw milk and even some food supplements (protein powder, vitamin D, Omega-3, etc.).

Everything is a question of quantity, if you respect 80% of the main principles of the paleo diet, you will get excellent results. If you do not have enough to eat paleo, do not deprive yourself, do you serve something else that allows you to eat your fill. Do not disorganize, sharing in a group is part of the pleasures of life and therefore well-being. Having a beer or a glass of wine occasionally has never hurt anyone. Conversely, just because you put 2 cherry tomatoes among your fries and there are strawberries in this beautiful " strawberry " ice cream, does not mean that your meal will be balanced. You have understood, everything is a question of balance, be regular, consistent, it is the key.

Nutrition is at the forefront of a healthy body system, and among the most important in your daily life, it is the main lever towards progression and performance, so it must not be neglected or left to chance. It is a vital need that we repeat several times a day and of which your general form will depend completely. So you now know why the paleo regime is at the center of all discussions and in other areas such as health and well-being.

Chapter Three

The Origin of the Paleo Diet

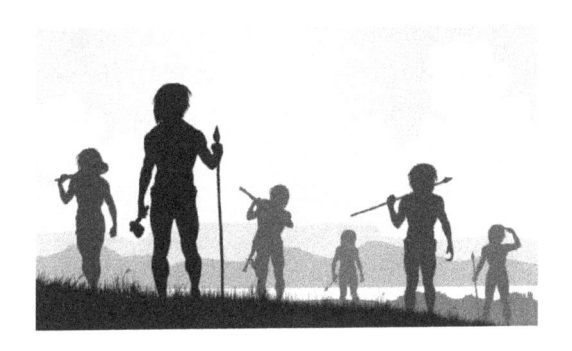

In ancient times, humans survived by hunting, fishing, and harvesting fruit, vegetables, and other products of the earth. This is why many scholars have called these our ancestors "hunter-gatherers". But it is not as immediate as it might seem. The variety of foods depended heavily on areas and seasons. And also by chance, skill and other factors that today would not be important or limiting at all. DNA research has shown that in the last 40,000 years, DNA has changed to a negligible percentage, quantifiable as only 0.02%, making, in fact, the constitution of man practically equal to that of men of the most recent Paleolithic that is Upper Paleolithic.

What Did They Eat?
It is done first to say what they did not eat or, better, what changed between 10,000 and 15,000 years ago (the period changes according to the areas considered). Between 10,000 and 15,000 years ago, a man began to understand that it was possible to avoid migrations linked to the alternation of the seasons and that it was possible to obtain conservable or usable food resources all year round. This possibility was linked to the

discovery and adoption of 2 new practices: agriculture and breeding.

Our eating habits and the decrease in physical activity play a decisive role in the emergence, at a pandemic level, of diseases called civilization, for example, coronary heart disease, hypertension, type 2 diabetes, and many others.

Surprisingly, these diseases are absent in the rare contemporary hunter-gatherer populations that have not yet come into contact with the western lifestyle. Their lifestyle seems not to have evolved since the Upper Paleolithic which is around 40,000 years ago.

Some researchers have associated this deplorable current situation with the rapid and frequent changes our environment has undergone for several decades. What is interesting is that unlike our environment and above all the food industry (and therefore of people's food), Our genome (our set of genes) has practically not changed. This leads us to say that socially, we are certainly in the 21st century, but genetically, we have remained in the Upper Paleolithic. Some believe it is this temporal gap between genome and environment that could explain the current rise in civilization diseases. We can partially associate the appearance and growing fame of the Paleolithic diet with these rather rational explanations.

However, not everyone agrees on the facts mentioned above, and numerous variables, as well as the evaluation of the context, must be taken into consideration.

If we take a step back in time, scientific literature reveals that the foods typically consumed during that era were ripe and sweet fruits, berries, meat, fish, crustaceans, insects, larvae, eggs, animal bone marrow, roots, tubers, nuts and seeds other than grasses. Strangely, this type of food provides about 25% of the energy intake of the typical person of our age. This means that now, most of our daily energy comes from seeds, dairy products, sugars, refined fats, and vegetables. On the other hand, the guidelines of some recognized institutions in the field of nutrition and the foundations of Paleolithic nutrition have several points in common. For example, take less sodium and refined sugars, along with a richer diet of fruit and vegetables.

The techniques used to reconstruct the typical paleo diet of the "ancient humans" are mainly based on the analysis of their teeth, but also the size and confirmation of their jaw. The exploration by anthropologists of the sites where our ancestors used to camp has made it possible to highlight the remains of animal bones and fish they have consumed, as well as the tools used to peel and prepare them. On the other hand, with the new technologies of microscopic dental analysis and chemical analysis techniques, we could have surprises about the variety of our ancestors' nutrition. Furthermore, the relationships between micronutrients (proteins, carbohydrates, and fats) found in their diet seem to vary depending on the historical sites studied and the methods of analysis used.

In addition, the paleo diet or 'evolutionary' diet is an urban legend launched for the first time by the gastroenterologist Walter Voegtlin (The Stone Age Diet, 1975), and taken up in the following years by various authors with studies of a scientific nature. The widely shared narrative indicates that the man would have regulated his genetic heritage, and therefore his physiology, eating mainly lean meat and vegetables during the Paleolithic (period ranging from 2.5 million to 10 thousand years ago). With the advent of agriculture and breeding, and the massive introduction of new foods such as cereals, milk, and derivatives, man would not have succeeded in adapting. Hence the development of diseases typical of civilization, such as obesity, diabetes and tooth decay.

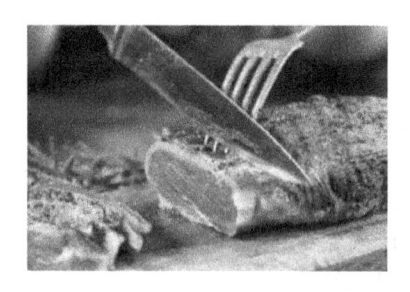

In reality, we do not know how our ancestors ate 1-2 million years ago in the various continents, in different seasons and latitudes. There were probably many 'paleo diets' that varied with the seasons. So we are talking about a food model that existed during our ancestral period.

Since the 1950s, the idea had spread among several anthropologists and even at the popular level, that the evolutionary step of Homo erectus would not be due to the consumption of tubers (some varieties of potatoes), but to the introduction in the diet of the meat (' Man the Hunter hypothesis '). The carcasses of numerous animals found in some caves would confirm this thesis. Unfortunately, the tubers or other vegetable products, being devoid of bones, have left no trace in the evolution of our species.

Several experts since the 1970s have considered this hypothesis a mere conjecture and recent analyses of the dental plaque of remains of Australopithecus sediba (South Africa, 2 million years ago) show that food was very similar to that of many contemporary primates. Nothing to do, therefore, with the supposed diet rich in meat so dear to the followers of the paleo regime.

Furthermore, residues of starch from different types of cereal grains found in archaeological sites 30,000 years ago in some part of the world like Russia, Italy, and the Czech Republic have been found. Therefore, a man introduced cereal starch into his diet long before 10 thousand years ago. Always the analysis of the dental plaque of Neanderthal man (200 thousand-40 thousand years ago) highlights the consumption of foods rich in gelatinized starch, a transformation that takes place only when starchy cereals are cooked.

Without disturbing the paleo nutrition experts, we can safely say that man has never eaten so much meat different from that of the Paleolithic as in recent decades, simply because there were no farms and it was not easy to get hold of it. Moreover, it was easily perishable because the cold chain did not exist, in a word, the refrigerator! Actually, we do not know what has led to the evolution which led to ' H homo sapiens brains of 1,300 cubic centimeters.

The ability to transform food before eating it (a sort of 'pre-digestion'), according to anthropologist Katharine Milton, and the introduction of fire to cook food, according to primatologist Richard Wrangham, have certainly helped to cope with the increased energy demands of the brain. Cooking is able to make perfectly assimilable foods that are not digestible let's think for example of a tuber or a raw potato, practically indigestible. It is not clear at which time the fire was used for cooking food, but some findings suggest 1.7 million years ago.

It is therefore not necessary to look at prehistory (paleo nutrition) to understand what is the ideal diet for humans, since we already know what the best food model is for living long and healthy: a diet based mainly on products of plant origin (plant-based diet) with plenty of cereals or tubers, fruit, vegetables, legumes, nuts, and small amounts of food of animal origin (meat, milk and derivatives, eggs, fish) or Mediterranean diets and vegetarian diets. The scientific evidence is consistent. The science of nutrition also tells us that it is good to avoid highly processed foods from the food industry in order to limit as much as possible the added sugars (sucrose, glucose, fructose, etc.), salt, fats (which increase density food calories) and alcohol (wine, beer, spirits).

Chapter Four

Advantages and Disadvantages of the Paleo Diet

The Paleo diet, also known as the Paleolithic diet or the cave diet, is a diet based on the type of diet that characterized the cavemen who lived some thousands years ago when, before advent of agriculture, human beings fed on the food obtained from practices such as hunting, fishing and harvesting the fruits of the earth that arose spontaneously. According to the proponents of the paleo diet, the human genome has practically not changed since then, while the advent of agriculture has substantially modified the diet of man, causing the health problems that today have exploded: obesity, overweight, diabetes, intolerances, allergies, and many others.

The paleo diet is therefore mainly protein based on the consumption of meat, fish, non-starchy vegetables, fruit, and nuts. The reasons behind the diet lie in the fact that when the Paleolithic age was nourished in this way the risk of running into serious pathologies was quite reduced and in fact the spread of cardiovascular, cancer and metabolic pathologies is strongly related to nutrition modern based on sugars, refined cereals, and junk food.

It should be noted that these foods should be chosen organic and as far as meat is concerned, since the one normally sold is meat stuffed with hormones, it should be consumed grass fed, the meat of cattle fed on grass and not on grains and hormones. The Paleo diet encourages eating less processed foods and more fruits and vegetables. It reduces the consumption of high-calorie foods by reducing the calorie intake and helping you lose weight.

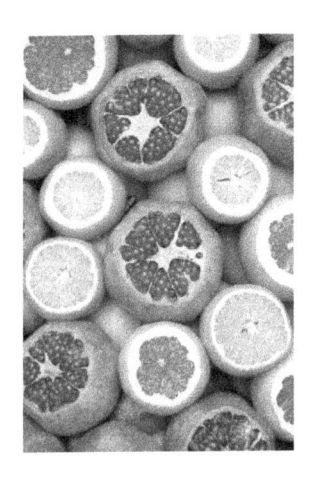

The diet is simple and does not involve counting calories. Some programs start from the "80/20" rule, so, for example, you will get 99% of the benefits if you manage to follow 80% of the time. This flexibility can make the diet easier to deal with, thus making it more likely to succeed.

The fiber intake also helps intestinal transit. The diet provides, for the necessary intake of carbohydrates and sugars, an important consumption of fruit and vegetables, precious sources of vitamins, antioxidants and mineral salts.

The paleo diet can be followed almost everywhere because all foods to eat are readily available. The paleo diet would reduce the level of insulin in the blood, but also cholesterol. The high consumption of fruits and vegetables also has health benefits since it provides multiple vitamins and minerals necessary for the proper functioning of the body.

Among the benefits of the paleo diet, we find the consumption of proteins, which quickly satiate and allow high-intensity physical activities. Another pro is definitely to take a break from all the industrial products we eat when we're in a hurry, or we're bored. No snacks, drinks, ready meals and junk foods. The health of the heart and the liver will certainly benefit.

So What Are the Disadvantage Sides of the Paleo Diet?
Undoubtedly positive is the preference for carbohydrates (albeit with many limitations) with low glycemic content and high fiber content. This allows you to lower the glycemic index and lose weight naturally.

On the other hand, milk and its derivatives are not included in the diet, and therefore, according to Paleo diet detractors, the necessary calcium and vitamin D intake is lacking. Furthermore, it is not always easy, nowadays and considering the development of society and consumption, find meat and fish that are not " treated."

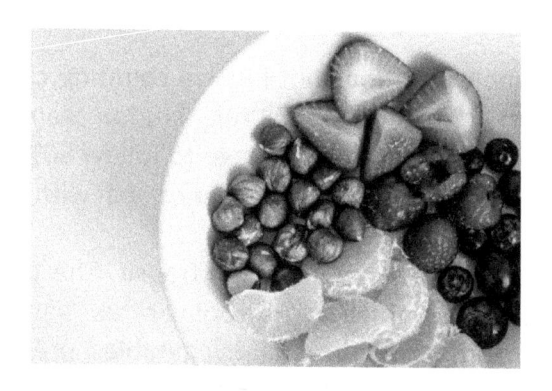

If the Paleolithic diet could have made sense two million years ago it is currently much more difficult to follow it to the letter; it provides for many restrictions, such as the lack of all leavened products, starchy foods, baked goods.

Furthermore, the consumption of mainly raw meat or game does not fall within the tastes of everyone, it is not easy to adapt to the flavor of raw meat or game, not to mention the difficulty nowadays of finding fresh meat suitable to eat raw without the risk to find health damage due to bacterial or parasitic contamination.

We must not forget that primitive man did not at all have a sedentary life: to burn all the fats (30-60%) required by the diet, you need to do some exercise, forget for a while the slippers and the sofa and dedicate at least 30 minutes a day to intense physical activity.

Several nutritionists claim that the Paleo diet is too restrictive and lacking in logic as it excludes whole categories of food by basing consumption on other categories. This way of eating is not balanced and, among other things, there is no scientific basis, according to experts, for which the followers of the Paleo live longer than others or are rarely subject to the onset of some diseases.

The Paleo diet must, however, be adapted to the different needs and if on the one hand, it may seem simple to do alone, on the other it is better to rely on an expert who can follow in the dietary path, especially if there are particular health conditions.

Like any other diet, the Paleolithic diet also shows some disadvantages. There are also some contraindications of the paleo diet. One of the risks is the yo-yo effect: the rapid weight loss in the first weeks and the subsequent vitamin D deficiency.

Like any other weight loss diet, the Paleolithic diet also has a list of permitted and prohibited foods which include:

- Foods permitted in the paleo diet: fruit, vegetables, red meat, white meat, eggs, fish
- Foods prohibited in the paleo diet: legumes, cereals, dairy products, foods with preservatives, sugars
- **Foods to be consumed in moderation: oil, tea, café, dried fruit**

However, as summer approaches, the desire to feel more beautiful, fit and ready to lose those extra pounds that winter has unfortunately given us is growing. To our rescue, large groups of food experts arrive ready to give us some tips to help us lose weight and finally feel in harmony with the warm season and with ourselves. One of the most popular diets in recent times is the Paleo diet, which refers to the typical diet of the Paleolithic men when neither agriculture nor livestock existed. Disadvantages of the Paleo Diet, meat and fish at will but. In those faraway times, men used to feed themselves with what, thanks to hunting and fishing, Mother Nature put at their disposal: mainly, therefore, meat and fish. Transposed in our times, the paleo diet certainly does not lend itself to being suitable for vegetarians by providing a large consumption of meat and fish in contrast to some of the most current trends that instead advise against the use of them, especially meat.

Another disadvantage of the Paleo diet, nutritional deficiencies banned from the Paleo diet dairy products and whole grains that normally today are part of a healthy and balanced diet. Furthermore, one of the most obvious disadvantages of the paleo diet is that it can prove to be expensive, especially due to the fact that being high in protein, cuts of meat can cost quite a bit. All artificial foods and artificial sweet substances are banned from the paleo diet, with the exception of honey, which must, however, be consumed in moderate quantities. Excluding basic food groups, the risk of nutritional deficiencies increases, which could be expected to compensate by taking food supplements and vitamins.

In addition, there are no accurate records of the diet followed by our Stone Age ancestors, so the Paleo diet is based on hypotheses, and its health claims have no scientific evidence. Most versions of the diet encourage large amounts of meat, which is in contrast to current evidence that discourages consumption.

Many versions prohibit dairy products and whole grains, which instead are part of a healthy and balanced diet. Like all high protein diets, Paleo can be expensive, depending on your choice of meat cuts. It is impossible to do the diet without eating meat, fish or eggs, so it is not for vegetarians.

Most versions of the Paleo Diet exclude basic food groups, increasing the risk of nutritional deficiencies unless careful substitutions are made. Use of food supplements is not excluded. The diet has some positive aspects, so an adapted version that does not prohibit food groups such as whole grains, dairy products and legumes could be a better choice.

This regime requires great rigor because it is very restrictive. Some foods such as bread, pasta, rice, and all other grain products can be difficult to remove from the diet because they are ubiquitous in our society. In addition, this diet can cause a yo-yo effect because of the rapid weight loss that occurs during the first two weeks. Also, this diet can cause deficiencies, but also bring saturated lipids into the body because of the overconsumption of meat and fish. In fact, farmed meat does not have the same nutritional qualities as a game consumed in the Paleolithic era.

However, by consuming foods in accordance with our genetic heritage, we, therefore, lower the risk of getting seriously ill. It would, therefore, be sufficient to replace sugar, cereals, bread, and pasta with meat, fish, fruit, roots, vegetables, and nuts.

Chapter Five

Foods And Common Mistakes You Must Not Consider When On The Paleo Diet

Did you start the paleo diet but you still don't feel as good as you would like? Are you struggling to digest? Not resting well and enough?

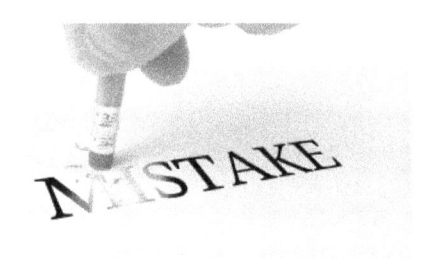

The following are Foods and Common Mistakes You Must not consider When on the Paleo Diet:
CONSUMING TOO MUCH FRUIT BECAUSE IT IS NATURAL FOOD
When we adopt a new diet that we consider healthy, many of us make the mistake of replacing junk food with industrial quantities of fruit, juices, and juices every hour of the day. The fact that fruit grows on trees does not mean that eating it continuously is always a good idea.
The fruit is more or less rich in fructose, which in large quantities causes inflammation, insulin response, and fat accumulation. Obviously, we are not talking about moderate amounts of low glycemic index fruit at meals or as snacks in active and metabolically healthy people. But for all the others, it is good to

remember that the fruit contains sugar. And as such it should be handled with care.

BELIEVING THAT FRUIT JUICES ARE HEALTHY

Fruit juices are often perceived as healthy, maybe it's because they come from fruit, right? Well, not always. Often (to be optimistic) commercial fruit juices are added with sugars and sweeteners of all kinds. It may also be that the juice does not contain any fruit, but only water, sugar, and some chemical fruit smelling concoction. But even if you can drink 100% real juices, you shouldn't drink juice (or at least not so much). The whole fruit contains some sugar, but it is linked to fiber, which slows the release of sugar in the blood. While fruit juice is different. It contains no fiber, no resistance to chewing and nothing to prevent us from swallowing massive amounts of sugar in a few seconds.

A cup of orange juice contains about two orange sugar. And the sugar contained in commercial juices is very similar to sugary drinks like Coca-Cola. So, eat whole fruit, and avoid fruit juices if you are trying to lose weight or have metabolic problems.

HOPE TO LOSE 20 KG. IN A WEEK

Seeing people feeling disappointed who after a week of paleo diet didn't lose enough weight. Of course, you will need to be patient. Since there is no healthy and sustainable diet in the world, in the long run, you lose all the extra pounds in weeks. For that, do the minestrone diet. But then, after a few weeks, you will have a hunger crisis and eat the whole fridge.

INCREASE WITH THE CONSUMPTION OF SEEDS AND NUTS

Nuts and seeds are absolutely part of the paleo diet. But they are rich in calories and above all contain quantities of polyunsaturated fats. In particular, omega-6, of which we are already quite supplied by consuming products of animal origin. Especially if these products come from animals raised in an unethical way and fed with soy and cereals.

The other problem is the anti-nutrients contained in these foods. Specifically, phytic acid. This substance is found in most plants, especially in the shell of the wheat, in the nuts and the seeds. It acts as a protection against insects, birds and other external agents. And although it is digested by cows and sheep, it is not digestible for humans.

Phytic acid binds to minerals (especially iron and zinc) in foods, preventing their absorption. It also interferes with the enzymes needed to digest food, such as pepsin (protein), amylase (starch) and trypsin (proteins in the small intestine). There is no official indication, but it appears that an amount between 100 to 400 mg per day is tolerable. To get an idea, 100 grams of almonds contain 1300 mg of phytic acid. However, there is a fairly simple way to reduce phytic acid in nuts and seeds.
AFRAID OF FAT

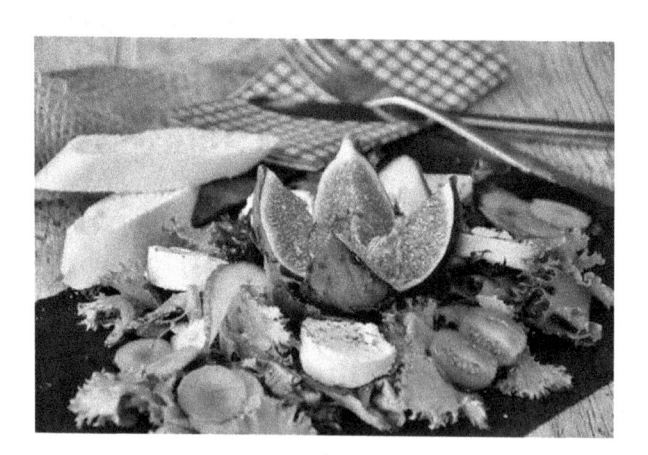

It is not surprising that after decades of propaganda, many people are still afraid of fat. Despite the deepening and understanding of the paleo principles, when we talk about fats, many people are still wary and take fat off the meat or cook as little oil as possible. Often with disastrous results, and with low-calorie diets, low in fat and carbohydrates. Then maybe they develop hypothyroidism and take it with the Paleolithic diet.

THINK THAT FATTY FOODS MAKE YOU FAT

It seems intuitive to deduce that eating fat makes you fat. For the simple fact that the thing that collects under the skin and that makes us look soft and chubby is called fat. So eating fat should make us even fatter. But it's not that simple. Although 1 gram of fat has more calories than 1 gram of carbohydrates or protein, high-fat diets don't make people fat. And as with all things, it depends on the context. A diet high in fat and carbohydrates at the same time will make you fat, but not because of fat. In fact, diets rich in fat (and low in carbohydrates) cause a greater loss of fat than diets that are low in fat

BELIEVING THAT SATURATED FATS HURT

Some tens of years ago it was decided that the heart disease epidemic was caused by the consumption of too much fat, and in particular, by saturated fat. This decision was based on studies and political choices, today considered and proven to be completely wrong.

An impressive review published in 2010 that considered 21 epidemiological studies with a total of 347,747 subjects led to the following results: no association between saturated fat and heart disease. The idea that saturated fats increased the risk of heart attack is an unproven theory that somehow became a popular belief.

While it is established that consuming saturated fats increases the amount of HDL (good cholesterol) in the blood and changes the consistency of LDL cholesterol particles, from small and dense (dangerous) to large and soft (harmless).

CONSUMING THE EGG WHITE AND THROW THE EGG YOLK

There is one thing that most nutritionists do with great success: demonizing incredibly healthy foods. The suspected number one are the eggs, which containing amounts of cholesterol are considered responsible for the increased risk of heart disease.

But recently it has been proven that cholesterol in the diet does not increase blood cholesterol. In fact, eggs primarily increase good cholesterol and are not associated with an increase in heart disease.

What remains is that eggs are one of the most nutritious foods that exist in nature. They are rich (especially the yolk) in every type of nutrient together with unique antioxidants that protect our eyes.

DON'T CONSUME ENOUGH CALORIES

When you eat real food, calories are a direct marker of nutrition. If you consume more calories from healthy food, it is wise to assume that you are also getting more nutrients. If you suffer from adrenal or thyroid problems, it may be more difficult to stabilize your blood sugar with fewer calories. Studies show that a low-calorie diet can cause a decrease in thyroid function or that it reduces its production of thyroid hormones.

To have a healthy metabolism, you need to make sure that you are consuming enough calories for your metabolic needs. This is mainly important for people who have already been diagnosed with adrenal and thyroid conditions. Low-calorie diets can also lead to hypoglycemia which can cause cortisol and insulin spikes.

TRYING TO PREPARE ANY DISH IN PALEO SAUCE

When you meet new vegetarians, they are usually interested in finding meat substitute foods for all the foods they abandoned with the new diet. So they consume hot dogs, sausages and other industrialized and often quite disgusting foods.

And the same thing happens to many Paleo diet newbies. They try to Paleolithic any food. This does not mean that we cannot occasionally give ourselves some paleo muffins, but as long as it does not become the rule in our diet.

Although these same contain paleo ingredients, they can contribute significantly to glycemic peaks or accentuate certain problems, especially in the presence of autoimmune conditions, bearing in mind that very often, in these recipes are considered large quantities of foods like nuts, seeds, and eggs. All foods that do not get along with autoimmune diseases and gastrointestinal problems.

IGNORING THE NUMBER OF PORTIONS

Despite what people say, calories do matter. And it is not true that by following the paleo diet you can eat when and how much you want. Especially if you are overweight and intend to lose weight. The inability to lose weight depends on various factors, but one of them certainly depends on the foods you choose. And for simplicity, especially when you are hungry and in a hurry, nuts and fruit seem to be the perfect combination. Maybe with a tablespoon of coconut butter. Let me be clear, these are perfectly paleo foods, but to be used with care and according to the objectives.

EAT LOTS OF SMALL MEALS DURING THE DAY

The idea that you have to eat so many small meals throughout the day to keep your metabolism active is a myth that makes no sense. It is true that eating increases the metabolism slightly during the digestive phase, but it is the total amount of food that determines the energy used, and not the number of meals.

Controlled studies where a group consumed many small meals and another group the same amount of food in fewer meals show that there is no difference between the two groups. In fact, a study conducted on obese subjects revealed that consuming 6 meals a day caused less sensation of satiety compared to 3 meals a day.

Not only is eating often useless in most people, but it can also be counterproductive. It is not natural for the human body to be continuously in a state of nourishment. Our ancestors used to fast from time to time and certainly did not eat the amount of food we consume today (in addition to quality, of course). When we do not eat for a prolonged period, a cellular process called autophagy cleans up the waste products from our cells.

Therefore, there is no evidence to show that consuming many small meals during the day is better than a few and more abundant meals. Not eating from time to time is good. If you have adrenal or glycemic problems, that's another story. And fasting is not for you then.

DO NOT EXPOSE YOURSELF TO THE SUN

Week after week, studies that confirm the importance of vitamin D increase. Despite this, many people avoid getting exposed to the sun and are covered with sunscreen for the sole pronunciation of the word sun. Why?

DO NOT COOK

It is impossible to follow the paleo diet without cooking. By doing so, you will not get results, and you will tire very soon. We are not talking about who knows what preparations. But if you plan to do your shopping once in a while and don't devote yourself to preparing your dishes, you'll flop.

We are talking about very simple things, like making a salad, cooking meat, fish and eggs and choosing fruit. And if you've been a world champion in pizza slices, restaurants, and frozen foods, you'll need a lot of discipline in the beginning. But your efforts will be amply repaid in all respects.

DO NOT DO PHYSICAL ACTIVITY

Sport is an important part of the Paleo style. If nutrition is a fundamental part, the importance of being physically active and lifting heavy loads from time to time should not be ignored. Paleo is not just a diet.

AVOID CARBOHYDRATES AT ALL COSTS AND FOR NO REASON

Many people who start paleo are attracted by the idea of losing weight fast while following a low-carb diet based on steak, eggs, avocado and coconut oil. If a low-carbohydrate diet can have therapeutic effects in some people, such as those with significant digestive problems, diabetes or diseases affecting cognitive function, there are many people who unnecessarily follow a low-carb or ketogenic paleo for the simple fact that they have been led to believe that nobody needs carbohydrates and that eating them will lead to disastrous health conditions. Many of these people are quite active, with intense workouts almost every day of the week. And this is not a good idea.

A perfect rule is not there, but if you are fickle, in perpetual lethargy, you are gaining weight despite the paleo, and you do not feel good as you would like with a paleo low-carb diet, you may find refreshment by increasing your carbohydrate consumption and improving your diet. Symptoms that you developed following an excessively low-carb diet.

EATING THE WRONG VEGETABLES

This recommendation is aimed primarily at people who have adopted a paleo diet due to digestive problems. For many people, paleo nutrition produces excellent digestive results. Eliminating cereals, dairy products and legumes can in many cases be enough to restore proper digestive function. But not for everyone. And some people, despite the paleo, don't solve their problems. Or even worse with paleo. Why? You may not be consuming enough carbohydrates to stimulate bowel movements. This could be due to a reduction in bowel function or the loss of healthy bacteria in the intestine (parasites). Or, especially in the presence of inflammatory diseases affecting the intestine, perhaps you are eating too many vegetables. The wrong kind. In particular, those vegetables rich in nature.

That is some types of carbohydrates that can feed certain classes of bacteria. In a healthy person, this is an absolutely positive thing. We feed healthy bacteria and protect ourselves from infections. In people with intestinal problems, it is possible that we are in the presence of an overgrowth of pathogenic bacteria. If this is the case, consuming universally healthy foods like apples and Brussels sprouts can create considerable stress and make us feel like a rag.

THINKING THAT BEING THIN IS EQUIVALENT TO BEING HEALTHY

Although it is always better not to be overweight, to be thin or to look fit does not mean that everything works perfectly inside. It is absolutely possible to be thin and diabetic. Being thin and getting a heart attack. Being thin and getting sick of any other disease. The external image is not everything. But not even remotely. This is a cultural, often disastrous illusion.

USE SUPPLEMENTS TO REMEDY BAD HABITS

Remember that companies that produce vitamins and supplements are also profit-oriented entities. Many people like to believe they can eat any crap, remedying this bad habit with some supplement. There is no such thing. Supplements are only supplements. They can be a powerful and very useful addition to a healthy diet, but they can never be a substitute for a healthy diet.

BELIEVING OUR DESTINY IS ALREADY WRITTEN IN OUR GENES

Even by the standards of the most conservative geneticists, we have control of our genetic expression between 80 and 97%. We all have dormant genes for anything, good or bad. You are not fat because your mother and father were fat. Nor are you destined to have a heart attack just because half of the people in your family have had one. And so on for diabetes, multiple sclerosis, and other diseases.

Genetics can certainly have some influence, but genes are turned on and off by regulatory genes, and regulatory genes are controlled primarily by nutrients. A gene will not express itself unless the internal environment favors its expression. And we have maximum control over this through the foods we eat, the emotions we experience, the toxicity of the environment in which we live and the lifestyle we choose to follow.

THINKING THAT A VEGAN DIET IS MORE "NATURAL"

All of us, regardless of our ideologies, ethnicity or religion, are genetically hunter-gatherers and 99.99% identical to our ancestors lived from 40,000 to 100,000 years ago. We are, in effect, creatures of the ice age, designed to consume a diet rich in foods of animal origin and natural fats, along with a variety of vegetable fiber.

Vegetarianism and veganism are modern ideas based more on ideological principles than on principles of human physiology and anthropological evidence.

Foods from animal sources are as healthy as their source, and no one should eat meat from animals raised in an unethical way, fed on cereals and forced to undergo hormonal treatments and antibiotics.

The alternative is not to be vegetarian or vegan. The alternative is to find foods derived from healthily raised animals. Plant foods are excellent, and a source of many antioxidants and phytonutrients, needed today more than ever. But these alone are far from being all we need to live healthily.

BELIEVING THAT FOLLOWING, THE PALEO DIET IS TOO EXPENSIVE

Nothing is further from reality. With a little organization, you can save money compared to a "normal" diet. Not to mention the money we will eventually save to go to the doctor when we are very "big."

GIVING IN TO THE IDEA OF EVERYTHING OR NOTHING

The typical worry of those who start paleo: can I do paleo diet even if I have a tight budget and can't afford grass-fed meat, organic vegetables and fruits?

The short answer is: yes.

And the mistake many newcomers make is to abandon the paleo because their budget does not allow them to always choose the best option. In case, if choosing the best products is not always possible, here are some practical tips:

1. *if you buy non-grass-fed meat, choose lean cuts. And it eliminates the visible fat before cooking.*
2. *if you can buy organic vegetables and fruits, choose the one you would eat with peel (apples instead of oranges, for example).*
3. Limit paleo sweets that often require the use of rather expensive flours.

BUNCHING ON LOW-FAT AND LOW-CARB PROTEIN

Reviewing your diet often matches the reduction of carbohydrate consumption (these vary from person to person).

What often happens is that people who choose to follow a low-carb regime do not eat enough fat, filling their plates with protein foods. So you often end up eating salads with a teaspoon of olive oil and unheard of chicken. This is the classic way to hurt yourself.

In the end, we are consuming a low-carb and even low-fat, but excessively high in protein diet. For those who choose a low-carb approach, it is appropriate to increase fat consumption and reduce protein consumption, with more or less reduced amounts of carbohydrates (depending on the objectives and physical activity).

ELIMINATE GLUTEN BUT EAT GLUTEN-FREE PACKAGED FOODS

You have decided to abandon the cereals, but then you have chosen a gluten-free diet. Excellent decision, but eating gluten-free bread is not ideal. Most (not to say all) of gluten-free sandwiches, pizzas, and desserts undergo major industrial changes and contain very low-quality vegetable oils (always to be avoided) and preservatives. In addition to having a noticeable glycemic impact, which is not what we hope for in most cases with a paleo diet.

REPLACE BARREL SUGAR WITH HONEY AND AGAVE JUICE

You have decided to eliminate the sugar, but the desire for sugar has not yet gone. So switch to "healthy" sweeteners like honey and agave juice. Agave is based on fructose and will not make you a nice long-term service. Honey, which contains less fructose than agave juice, should be used sparingly. Especially if you're trying to lose weight. The best alternative is to resist, integrating with a bit of glutamine and eventually, use a little stevia, waiting for the adaptation step to pass and your body learns to use the new fuel at its best.

ASK YOURSELF ANY PALEO QUESTION

There are people who want to see whatever happens in their lives through the Paleolithic lens. Computers and modern medicine did not exist in the Paleolithic era. So, shouldn't we use them? It could also be so, but we have the benefit of modern science and research to combine with the paleo diet, to get the best possible results, and it would be unreasonable not to make use of the opportunity.

DON'T LEAVE YOUR BODY TIME TO ADAPT

Sometimes the body needs some time, especially if you are experiencing chronic discomfort. Take all the time you need.

ABANDON THE DIET BECAUSE YOU ARE LOSING TOO MUCH WEIGHT

Did you start the paleo diet and you were skinny? And are you continuing to lose weight? So you decide to go back to old habits. It happens, but there could be a problem like an excess of intestinal permeability with relative malabsorption. Or you are simply not eating enough. Consume a lot, and maybe you do intense physical activity. You can increase the amount of fat. Or carbohydrates like fruit. Or add starches like potatoes.

CHECK CONTINUOUSLY

It is important to be aware of your state of health. A person who is well, will not notice particular variations in his well-being, but in the presence of pathological conditions such as inflammatory or autoimmune diseases, the speech changes. And even a single piece of bread or a glass of milk could restart the inflammatory process and bring you back to a state of chaos. So if you resist early on, it is very likely that you will no longer have any remorse or desire to consume old foods.

BELIEVING THAT THE PALEO DIET IS JUST A DIET

Paleo is a holistic lifestyle that includes nutrition but also other factors such as exercise, sleep and stress management. If you cannot recognize sleep as a key component of your health, you are forgetting an essential ingredient. Sleep assists you in the regulation of weight, stress, hormones, and metabolism.

NOT SLEEPING WELL AND ENOUGH

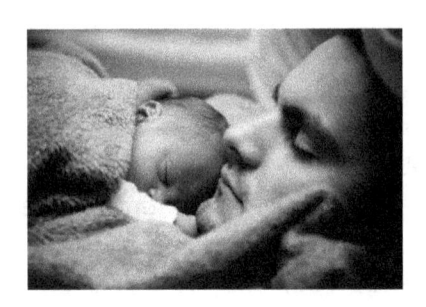

Sleeping is an essential part of a healthy lifestyle, and it is probably the most important factor. Without adequate sleep, you can follow a perfect paleo diet along with a fitness regimen, but you will never achieve the best shape. Without getting enough sleep, your body does not work properly, it does not fully recover after physical activity, and you find it difficult to keep stress under control. Finding out why you are not sleeping like you should and trying to understand the reasons and solve them is a necessary step to improve your health.

CONSUME FOODS TOO RICH OF AGES

AGEs stand for Advanced glycation end-products. That is compounds that are naturally formed in the body by the chemical reaction between sugars and proteins. If the concentration of AGEs in the blood becomes excessive, these final products can cause damage to almost any tissue and organ in our body. In practice, they act to permanently activate low-grade inflammation by binding to cellular receptors known as RAGEs. These reactions, when excessive, appear to be associated with premature aging and most chronic diseases such as type 2 diabetes, Alzheimer's, autoimmune diseases, etc.

The good news is that for those who follow the Paleo diet, most of these problems are reduced. Fruits and vegetables, as well as eggs, are poor in AGEs. And also raw meat and fish. But it's not like we can always eat meat.

It is in fact when we cook meat and fish, which increases the formation of AGEs. And the worst way to do it is by cooking at high temperatures (embers, barbecues). Therefore, it is preferable to choose gentler cooking methods such as using the slow cooker, which minimizes the number of AGEs but still guarantees adequate cooking and gourmet flavors.

Chapter Six

Amazing ways to Incorporate the Paleo Diet into Your Lifestyle

If you've ever looked around for a diet program to help you lose a few inches, you've probably come across the Paleo diet. At first glance, it doesn't seem to be much about the Paleo diet, very popular, and low in carbohydrates, high in protein, and free of processed foods.

Making the transition from today's diet to that of our ancestors is not necessarily easy. Depending on what you expect from the paleo diet, your life situation and your ultimate goal (to stay in the paleo or not), you may have the interest to go gradually according to the Japanese method of small steps. We present here three gradual stages of the paleo diet, which can be adapted one after the other, depending on what you want.

It is, in short, a diet that eliminates all foods that have appeared since the Neolithic with the advent of agriculture (salt, sugar, dairy products, cereals, legumes but also refined oils). Why? Because if our DNA has remained the same since the Paleolithic, our diet has changed radically from that time and much more since the industrial revolution. The food that we are adapted to, that which allows us to be the fittest and healthy, would be that of the Paleolithic: fresh food from hunting or gathering (meat, fish, poultry, eggs, vegetables and fruits, nuts and seeds, herbs and spices). Exit the baguette, lentils, cheese and all industrial foods.

It's a no-brainer that our caveman ancestors don't have a lot of food choices back in the day. As such, you are only allowed to feed on grass meat, fish, fruit, vegetables, eggs, nuts and seeds, and some oils (olive, nuts, flax seeds, macadamia nuts, avocado, coconut).

This means that things like cereals, legumes, refined sugar, dairy products, refined vegetable oils, processed foods, and even salt are off-limits. It is rare, however, to eat three non-Paleo meals a week. So in theory, you should be able to indulge in the occasional beer or slice of pizza, right?

By eating what corresponds to the original functions of the organism, it is indeed reduced, but one could also prevent a number of diseases, especially those called civilization. Changing your diet is not easy. It is necessary, even for the most motivated ones, to face temporary discomfort and to unlearn food. That's why the specialists of this diet now propose to gradually follow the example of dietitian-nutritionist.

We will now offer you three progressive stages to move to the paleo, each in their way you will already do good. Sure you can go directly to the 3rd stage without passing through the square.

Step 1: The Basic Paleo

Aim: eliminate industrial foods, better choose others, say goodbye to gluten

At this point, it's all about better choosing your food. The big restriction is no longer eating gluten. Why start with him? Because a priori is the elimination of gluten that has the most beneficial effect on health. For bread, if you used to eat baguette or white bread and you cannot imagine life without, you can introduce an extra step of replacing your white bread with a whole loaf of bread or leavened cereals. And by decreasing as much as possible your portions.

Foods to avoid
- Cakes, buns, and pastries
- Industrial foods containing additives
- Alcoholic drinks containing gluten and sugar (beer, cocktails)
- Grain products (bread, pasta, biscuits)
- Legumes (soy, lentils, dried beans)
- **Sugar and sweets**

Authorized foods

- Meat, eggs, fish and other foods high in animal protein
- Good fats (olive oil, coconut oil, animal fat, avocado, butter)
- Vegetables, fruits, nuts, hazelnuts, almonds
- Herbs and spices
- Dairy products
- Dark chocolate with more than 70% cocoa, honey
- **Tea, coffee without sugar**

You usually eat Bread, Treats and industrial snacks, Sugar, legumes, Cereals with gluten (pasta, semolina, wheat, etc.), Sunflower oil,
Replace it with Paleo bread, buckwheat in all its forms, Chocolate with 90% cocoa, nuts, and raw seeds, Honey, Vegetables (sweet potato for example), Cereals without gluten (rice, quinoa, millet, buckwheat), Olive or coconut oil.

Step 2: The Classic Paleo

Aim: those of the basic paleo + end of dairy products and cereal products (even without gluten)

If you have not done it yet, it's time to say goodbye to bread. And also cheese, yogurt, and milk. For butter, it is possible to clarify it to extract lactose. Some Paleo authors maintain it at this stage arguing that it contains little lactose anyway.

Foods to avoid
- Cakes, buns, and pastries
- Industrial foods containing additives
- Alcoholic drinks containing gluten and sugar (beer, cocktails)
- Grain products (bread, pasta, biscuits)
- Legumes (soy, lentils, dried beans)
- Sugar and sweets
- Dairy products

Authorized foods
- Meat, eggs, fish and other foods high in animal protein
- Good fats (olive oil, coconut oil, animal fat, avocado, clarified butter)
- Vegetables, fruits, nuts, hazelnuts, almonds

- Herbs and spices
- Dark chocolate with more than 70% cocoa, honey
- Tea, coffee without sugar (but in limited quantity)

You usually eat Bread, Treats and industrial snacks, Sugar, legumes, Cereals, Sunflower oil, Tea and coffee, Milk.

Replace it with Paleo bread, Chocolate with 90% cocoa, nuts, and raw seeds, Honey, Vegetables (sweet potato for example), Nuts, natural seeds, Olive or coconut oil, Herbal tea, Coconut milk,

Step 3: The Strict Paleo

Aim: those of the classic paleo + elimination of alcohol, tea, coffee, and chocolate

At this point, you will only eat food from the supermarket's fresh aisle (or better, bought directly from farmers from the market). It is about consuming the most "raw" foods possible. More alcohol, more tea, coffee, chocolate. On the social level, it's more restrictive. This may require you to have your food at hand if you are invited.

If you are at this stage, it is most often because of strong personal conviction (ecological for example) or because of health disorders you have led there.

Foods to avoid

- Cakes, buns, and pastries
- Industrial foods
- Grain products (bread, pasta, biscuits)
- Legumes (soy, lentils, dried beans)
- Sugar and sweets
- Dairy products
- All alcohols
- Tea, coffee, dark chocolate

Authorized foods

- Meat, eggs, fish and other foods high in animal protein
- Good fats (olive oil, coconut oil, animal fat, avocado, clarified butter)

- Vegetables, fruits, nuts, hazelnuts, almonds
- Herbs and spices

You usually eat Bread, Treats and industrial snacks, Sugar, legumes, Cereals, Sunflower oil, Tea and coffee, Milk, Alcohol, Chocolate.

Replace it with Paleo bread, Chocolate with 90% cocoa, nuts, and raw seeds, Honey, Vegetables (sweet potato for example), Nuts, natural seeds, Olive or coconut oil, Herbal tea, Coconut milk, Water, Coconut Chips.

In any case, whatever the stage, to follow a paleo diet in the world today, it is better to keep in mind to eat Paleo 80% of your time and give yourself a 20% margin for outings, and invitations.

Chapter Seven

Time to Prepare Your Kitchen for the Paleo Diet

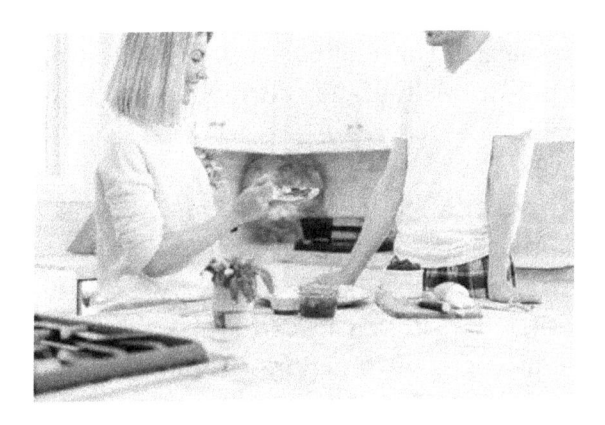

Preparing healthy and nutritious Paleo diet snacks in your kitchen is easier than it seems. Often we tend to consider the moment of the snack as a bad food habit, but in reality, it is we who do not know how to make good use of it. In fact, due to a bad food organization, most people (especially in the late afternoon, in work or study places) take refuge behind the display of a "junk food machine"; in the throes of hunger attacks.

Certainly, this does not mean to have a snack! At least not that healthy and dietetic snack contemplated by the Paleo diet. In all those cases it is obvious that this is not a good food habit. So the physiological problems will begin to be felt chronically, at least as chronic as the intake of these junk foods without nutrients and that affect human health.

Being able to choose, in these cases, it is preferable to avoid having a snack.

If you are also of this opinion but you are not going to go hungry, then this is for you! You'll find lots of interesting ideas to make your Paleo Snacks to take wherever and whenever you want. Easy to make and practical to carry, Paleo Snack fits perfectly with an authentic and natural lifestyle. It doesn't matter if you are a young girl, a student, a career woman, a family man or a pensioner who enjoys free time: with a bit of organization, you will be able to realize your healthy snacks in the hectic everyday life. Find out which healthy and nutritious snacks are right for you:

DRIED FRUIT MIX

Versatile and practical, dried fruit is an excellent food for snacking in all those moments and those days where you can't afford anything more than a jacket pocket. A real health pocket; in fact, the dried fruit is rich in cerebral active nutrients that improve general cognitive functions. A handful of dried fruit gives strength and energy precisely in those hours where fatigue begins to be felt.

If we now consider that dried fruit does not create halitosis problems and specifically almonds contribute to the natural whitening of teeth, without a doubt, we can consider it the Paleo Snack idea that is the smartest and most versatile of all. It is highly recommended not to overdo the quantities; the risk is to arrive at lunch or dinner, with a huge sense of satiety.

BOILED EGGS

A hard-boiled egg that is eaten in 2 bites.

Why not? Eggs are not only a fundamental ingredient for seasoning and filling a recipe, but they are also an excellent snack (practical and healthy) that can be enjoyed in the hectic everyday life. In reality, it is a question of having a bit of organization in the morning. Pause 30 seconds in the kitchen to boil the eggs before entering the shower, and you're done.

10 minutes later (for example the shower time) drain the boiled eggs and let them cool before placing them in the Tupperware. Furthermore, the eggs have a high level of conservation, and the shell protects them from any external contamination.

Let the eggs cool naturally and keep them in the fridge for a week if possible:
- You will have to remember to prepare your snack eggs 1, maximum 2 times a week.
- So the real difficulty lies in being able to consolidate new eating habits! Because otherwise an egg is eaten in 2 bites and its benefits are lasting.
- **Such a high level of protein (as many as 7 g) in so little food.**

Furthermore, egg proteins are vital because they contain essential amino acids and all in usable form; that is, those that the human body cannot produce on its own in a manner sufficient to satisfy the physical needs:
- Phenylalanine;
- isoleucine;
- Lysine;
- Leucine;
- Methionine;
- threonine;
- Tryptophan;
- **Valine.**

Eggs are considered by the medicine an essential food for pregnant women and during the lactation period:

The high level of choline (or Vitamin J, an essential coenzyme for the constitution of cell membranes) present in eggs, contributes to the healthy and rigorous development of the nervous system of the fetus and prevents it from congenital diseases.

Essential, natural, practical and long-lasting; boiled eggs are an excellent healthy snack, to be taken into consideration among the Paleo Snack ideas that can be enjoyed in the hectic everyday life.

WILD BERRY VARIETY
The colors of the forest in practical takeaway trays.

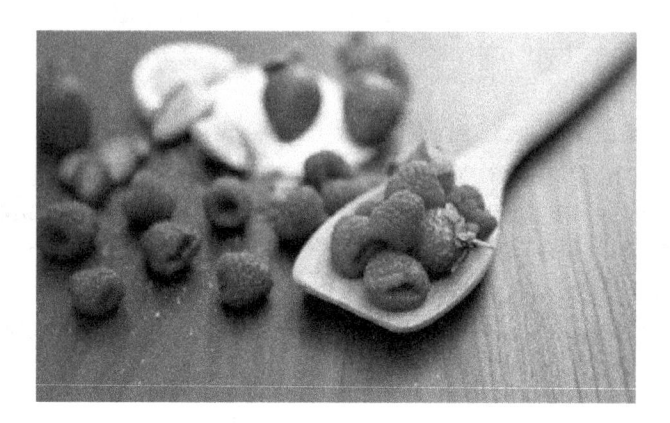

Fresh, colorful and of a thousand varieties the fruits of the undergrowth (precisely because they share their habitat despite having properties and distinctive characteristics between them) have invaded our food. Just stop in the nearest shop in the city to fill a bag of berries, to be enjoyed in peace during the workday; when hunger begins to strike.
In fact, berries (all fruit in general) is always recommended to take it away from meals in order to be able to synthesize as many vitamins (nutrients) as possible quickly, precisely when the intestine is not processing other foods. Excellent as essential to take out of meals; wild berries are a sweet healthy snack, to be taken into consideration among the Paleo Snack ideas that can be enjoyed in the hectic everyday life.
BANANA & APPLE

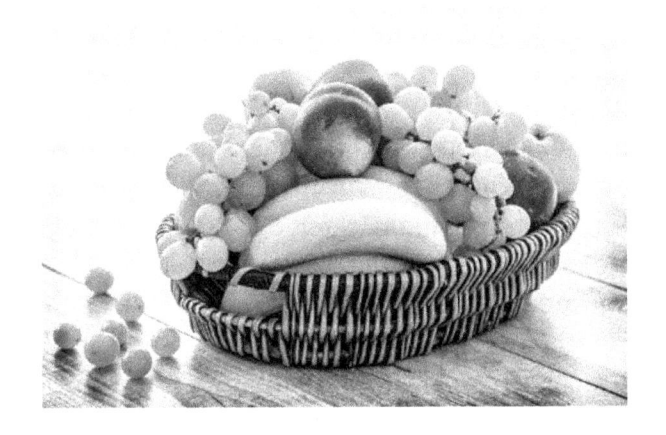

The choice is yours; apple or banana?
Banana and apple are the perfect combinations to alternate as an everyday snack. When the preparation gets out of hand, you can always look back and pick up an apple, or turn sideways and rip a banana out of its helmet.
"One day, apple, one day, banana ... you live for 100 years!"
DATES & PRUNES FROM CALIFORNIA
With dark color and a unique flavor: California plums.
Dried because it is dehydrated (i.e., released from all liquids) the California Plum and rich in nutrients, a true elixir of well-being. Already packaged, easy to find and with good preservation, the California plums and dried dates in effect acquire a place among the most comfortable and common Paleo Snack ideas to find. Real healthy snacks that reduce the sense of fatigue contribute to the health and shine of skin and hair.
Also California plums:
- they are very rich in copper, potassium, magnesium, vitamin B6 and K;
- contribute to the normal functioning of the digestive system;
- **they regulate and maintain the level of cholesterol in the blood.**

Superfoods! Go easy on the greed! Especially if you are on a Paleo diet. Dried fruit contains a medium or high GI (Glycemic Index)

THE DRIED MEAT

Fine meat rich in history. The dried meat fine as per tradition.

Nothing to do with other over-the-counter gourmet products, which in fact often contain carcinogenic preservatives (Nitrite and Nitrate) and other additives.

With rather modest origins, the dried meat has then conquered the food market as a niche product and quite delicious. In fact, originally the best cuts were intended for the consumption of fresh meat, while the less tender parts of the meat and the particularly adult meats were seasoned with salt and other spices (therefore: salted, dried and seasoned).

The main purpose of the poor people was to be able to satisfy the demand for meat all year round, and drying the meat was the only solution.

But when the needs of people are transformed into traditions, delicious techniques, short chain processes; the dried meat has known its true fame.

AVOCADO STUFFED WITH GUACAMOLE; INGENIOUS INVENTION

It takes no more than 10 minutes of preparation (just peel the avocado and crush it with lemon, oil, salt, pepper, and coriander). You can pour the cream into a small takeaway jar (airtight), which is then placed inside a larger Tupperware, so as to carry two carrots, a cucumber, and a knife to peel the vegetables in a single container.

The benefits of avocado are innumerable, in fact, rich in potassium and calcium; it is an essential food to maintain the health of the skin, hair, and brain. In addition, the avocado contains significant amounts of monounsaturated fats that prevent the risk of diabetes and defend the heart from cardiovascular diseases.

A, B1, B2, D, E, K, H, and PP are the innumerable vitamins present in a single fruit.

Maybe it doesn't represent the maximum in terms of practicality, but anyone in the nutrition world (Paleo or not Paleo) would recommend a nice pudding of avocado for a snack.

SELECTION OF OLIVES

Simple Olives, what could be more natural and authentic than making a snack by munching on so-called healthy fats? Olives certainly deserve a place among the Paleo Snack ideas that can be enjoyed in the hectic everyday life, even if the strong stimulating effect of the appetite must be pointed out.

Make sure you have at least 2 or 3 nuts in your drawer if you don't want to risk sinking your teeth into the desk from hunger.

CRUSHED ALMOND

Homemade organic almond crushed.

A puree with an explosive and enthralling taste, you won't be able to stop. To be jealously guarded in the secret drawer of our office, ready to pop out at the first event. Excellent accompanied with fruit; with the weighing of almonds, it is easy to transform a simple banana into a delicious Paleo Snack, which can be enjoyed as a snack in the hectic everyday life.

Almond cream is completely natural, with no added colorings, additives or palm oil. Not only is it not harmful to health but it also contains all the healthy properties of almond concentrated in an explosion of taste.

CRISPY ALGAE

Fine and crunchy algae, the favorite snack of the Japanese.

If you are a lover of sushi and oriental cuisine, your diet can only include an excellent and healthy snack based on crispy algae. Spreadable and toasted are a valid alternative to crackers and chips; with the incomparable difference that (in addition to not being harmful) algae act as a healthy remedy for various psychosomatic problems.

Rich in:
- minerals,
- vitamins (A, B, C, E, and K),
- fibers;

- **and in view of the great practicality in transport and consumption, crispy algae deserve a place among the Paleo Snack ideas, usable in the hectic everyday life.**

A HANDFUL OF SEEDS

Pocket and smart as the gesture of pulling the crumbs to the pigeons the seeds of:
- pumpkin,
- poppy,
- sunflower,
- sesame,
- linen,
- **they are an excellent natural hunger break with a very high nutritional value.**

The seed mix is a classic among the Paleo Snack ideas to propose in any circumstance.

ORGANIC COCONUT DRINK

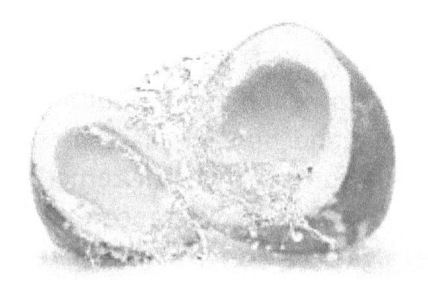

Pure coconut water directly from the fruit. Rich in fiber, enzymes, magnesium, and potassium, it also has the advantage of being naturally sweet (with no added sugar). It is said to be one of the beauty secrets of the great world stars. If you feel like a superstar, all you have to do is follow the wave of success and start sipping the elixir of youth too.

Superstars aside, the coconut organic drink is a great Paleo Snack idea to sip in the hectic everyday life.

Chapter Eight

Paleo Diet for Families with Kids

The philosophy of the Paleolithic diet is that the ideal diet corresponds to that of our ancestors. One of the greatest determinants of our nutritional needs is our genes. And since our genes have not changed (0.02%), that's why we should eat like our ancestors. The paleo diet, also known as the ancestral diet, therefore focuses on a diet low in carbohydrates but high in fiber and protein. Lean meats, poultry, fish and seafood, eggs, nuts and seeds, and low-starch fruits and vegetables (i.e., no potatoes, yams, etc.) are preferred. However, this diet excludes dairy products, grain products, legumes and salted or processed foods (canned goods, cakes, soft drinks, etc.).

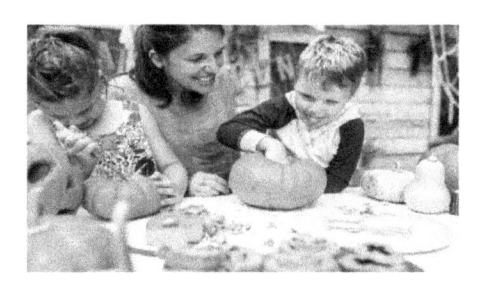

Nutrition in children and even more so nutrition education in children touches them because as a parent who has little kids, and you daily try to teach them what are the real foods, those of nature, and to consciously choose what to eat.

The problem of nutrition in children peeps out among new parents shortly after the birth of their young. In fact, after 5/6 months from birth, some pediatricians propose weaning and the insertion of the first baby food. Even if the nutrition of our children is correct, it begins even before birth, because they absorb the nutrients and anti-nutrients that mothers ingest, so we must think about eating at best even during the period of pregnancy.

Observing the rules of the Paleo diet in a family with children is quite easy until one is confronted with the outside world, therefore with the nursery school, the kindergarten, the birthday parties of the friends but also simply the gardens. In these places, your children will see other children eating things "different" from theirs. In your eyes they are junk, to them, they are something they have never seen, tasted, and surely they are intrigued.

For this reason, it is important to teach people to choose consciously and not feel obligated to make a choice because they said, mom and dad. This of course if there are no serious allergies or autoimmune diseases that require strict control of the food consumed by our children.

Some children at school eat exactly what other children eat (because some of them don't have any particular pathologies or allergies), but when some of them leave school they bring a fruit, or a paleo sweet, like paleo cookies or paleo muffins, and at breakfast and dinner instead they eat natural and unprocessed foods granted in the Paleo Diet. They are very fortunate because some of the school that these children attend is very attentive to food, to snack, centrifuges or extracts, and desserts are made daily and not packaged.

In any case, the best advice is to let your child taste everything, always at the clinical level, if possible, and make them choose what is good and what is not.

For example, that children easily realize the "damage" caused by "modern" food, another example is if they eat potato chips at a party, the next day or evening itself often has blisters in their mouth that burn them, or if they eat packaged ice cream the next day they have a blocked nose or another simple sign that we can teach them to recognize is the burning bottom. Children know very well that these little annoyances are due to what they ate and soon learn to adjust themselves.

The paleo diet is to feed only ingredients that our prehistoric ancestors had access. Meat, fish, fruits, vegetables, eggs, and nuts are at the heart of these recipes. This offers parents baby recipes based on this very special diet. According to doctors, this baby recipe contains ten times more vitamin A than the recommended daily intake for a toddler.

Today Paleo Diet is the right diet for families with kids, which can be very useful to mothers and fathers who always have little time. And then even being able to prepare dinner in no time can be very useful. The diet is a natural recipe for messy families and also enhance mental fitness for a kid, Paleo Diet aims to accompany families to discover a healthy, practical and enjoyable food style based on the prehistoric era.

In fact, how can a natural and healthy kitchen be combined with a family with limited time, in today's hectic life? This is the mission of " The Paleo Diet ", the diet for mothers and fathers with little time but with the desire to gather the family around a table to savor the taste of simple, healthy, and delicious recipes.

It also benefits the kids psychologically and gives parents the chance to show how to bring children closer to food and sheds light on some important aspects related to nutrition and health.

How to educate your children to an evolutionary diet?

As a parent you can personally follow the Paleo Diet when your kid is 1-year-old, so you can start the classic weaning following the rules dictated by the pediatrician, starting with the tapioca and vegetable broth, then introducing one vegetable at a time, then meat and fish. You may resort to homogenized glass only in cases of "emergency" such as long journeys or to prepare a meal on the fly at times of heavy workload.

Otherwise, you will have to always prepare the homogenized vegetables, meat, and fish, the vegetable and meat broth, obviously starting from the raw materials and not using nuts or preparations nor salt. It seems difficult and a great waste of time but with the assurance, you will need only a few minutes of effort to prepare large quantities of homogenized which you can keep in the freezer. In this way you can mix proteins and vegetables at will, always offering new tastes to the child and giving their palate and digestive system to new natural foods. Another factor not to be neglected in preparing homogenized at home is that as the baby grows, you can blend the preparation less and less and propose it to the baby so that he learns to chew properly and gradually.

However, on the subject of nutrition for families with children as a serene parent who does not force and does not oblige them to eat one thing rather than another. The best approach is teaching.

Chapter Nine

Paleo Diet: The Perfect Breakfast Ideas

Breakfast is one of the most important daily meals that should be consumed by the individual and never give up, because of its importance in strengthening the body and make it able to do his meals daily to the fullest. This meal is characterized by its ability to maintain the ideal weight of the individual; do not affect the weight in the case of a diet program, unlike lunch and dinner.

With its diet based exclusively on nature, the Paleo diet is ideal to benefit your body and lose weight. Here are all the keys to a successful Paleo breakfast.

The "Paleolithic" diet advocates a return to the diet of our ancestors, which has multiple health benefits. It consists of eating only a variety of fruits, vegetables, meats, eggs, and seeds, that is unprocessed foods. And recipes for feasting at breakfast time are not lacking.

If you like fruit, you will be able to indulge yourself with delicious meals with cottage cheese and berries or with tasty and crunchy fruit granola. To surprise your taste buds when you wake up, try our coconut pudding, chia seeds, and red berries. What a delight! And to hydrate you, you can sip succulent mango, apple, lemon, and honey smoothie.

If you're more of a foodie and savory, you should enjoy our paleo bread and our salty pistachio cookies. To fill up on protein, you can make an omelet with tomato or little eggs spinach casserole. Simple and really tasty recipes that only need a few ingredients.

The Paleo diet can also create ultra-gourmet recipes that will delight the taste buds as soon as you wake up. Paleo muffins made with applesauce and rice flour will suit the whole family. Bowl cake with oatmeal will allow you to refuel for the day. It is prepared in a jiffy, and you can decline it according to your tastes and your desires.

Paleo breakfast can be problematic for some people who go on a paleo diet. The paleo diet prohibits industrially manufactured foods. For example, you can eat red meat, but not processed meat.

Let's look at the foods that are allowed under a paleo diet: fruits, vegetables, meat, oils, and nuts. For each food category, you will find examples that you can include for your paleo breakfast.

Fruits

Fruits are prominent in the paleo breakfast. Want to lose weight? In this case, choose fruits low in sugar for breakfast. Examples of common low sugar fruits:

- grapes
- Watermelon
- blueberries
- **raspberries**

Vegetables

Vegetables are preferred for fruits. Indeed, vegetables are much lower in sugar. You can eat at will. On the other hand, do not eat fried vegetables. Although most people prefer fruit, vegetables are a good place for breakfast. Here are some vegetables that you can incorporate into your paleo breakfast.

- asparagus
- carrots
- **spinach**

Meat

People on a paleo diet are encouraged to focus on meat at breakfast. Proteins and lipids go hand in hand, and that goes for the Paleo breakfast. No other diet encourages the consumption of red meat at breakfast. Here are some types of meat that you can incorporate into a paleo breakfast.

- Chicken thighs
- Chicken breast
- Salmon
- **Lamb**

Oils

One might think that oils should be avoided as much as possible since they are very rich in fat. However, this is a mistake: it is mainly carbohydrates that make you fat. Oils and fats of natural origin are important for the body. Here are some oils you can add to your paleo breakfast to get more energy:
- Coconut oil
- Olive oil
- Avocado oil
- **Macadamia nut oil**

Nuts

Nuts are very good for health, but very caloric. Be especially careful with cashews. Peanuts are often considered nuts, wrongly. Better not to consume it. Here are some examples of nuts that will go well with a paleo breakfast.
- Almonds
- Hazelnut
- Pecan nuts
- **Nuts**

The paleo diet is a complex diet. It's about consuming what our ancestors ate. For most foods, this will not be a problem, but there are exceptions. In particular, you must not consume meat from animals that have been fed on cereals. Some foods are to be excluded because they did not exist in prehistoric times. These products do not fit the paleo way of life, and therefore have no place in the paleo breakfast. Here are some examples of foods to give up:
- Legumes - for example, black beans, and peanuts
- Cereals - for example, rye and brown rice
- Added sugar - for example, in cakes and sweets

- Almost all dairy products
- **Vegetable oils - for example, rapeseed oil and soybean oil**

Better a lot of fat than a lot of carbohydrates. Research has shown that it is better for you to consume a lot of fat than a lot of carbohydrates. Participants in one study were divided into two groups. One group was on a high carbohydrate diet and the other group on a high-fat diet. As a result, the group whose diet was high in fat lost more weight. The high-fat diet has also led to a drop in blood pressure and low cholesterol. This study is proof of the power of the paleo diet.

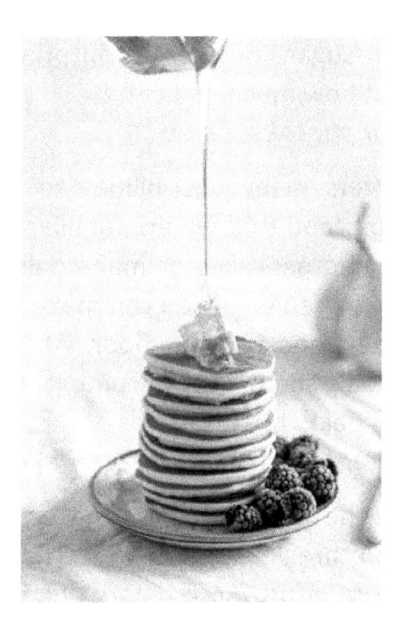

The Standard Breakfast Is Far Too Rich in Carbohydrates
Often, the breakfast we eat is way too rich in carbohydrates. The fault lies not only with bread but also with cereals. A paleo breakfast excludes this type of food. To make it easier to switch to a paleo diet, it is important to have breakfast that you like.

You do not want eggs or meat in the morning? No problem: there are many other solutions.

Ideas for A Perfect Paleo Breakfast

The difference between an ordinary dinner and a paleo dinner does not imply a drastic change. As part of the Paleo diet, the dinner poses a little problem when you think it is a diet. However, this is rarely the case with breakfast. Skip two slices of jam to a paleo breakfast is a big step. Here are some ideas to help you better appreciate your paleo breakfast.

1. *Stop Counting Calories*

With the paleo breakfast, no need to count the calories. Stick to the paleo recipes, and you'll lose weight fast. You can choose fruit depending on sugar content, but in principle, you do not have to think about how much you eat.

2. *Try the bread or pancakes paleo*

The paleo diet offers many possibilities to vary its diet, but sometimes we want food that we are familiar with. In this case, you can opt for paleo pancakes or make paleo bread, with all your favorite paleo ingredients. You can make crepes made from coconut milk, honey, and coconut flour. At first sight, making bread without cereals seems rather complicated, but there are dozens of delicious paleo bread recipes.

3. *Prepare your breakfast the day before*

Some bread from the bakery, a little butter, some jam and a glass of milk, and breakfast is ready! The paleo breakfast requires a little more effort. Accommodating the paleo diet in a busy life requires some changes. One idea is to prepare your dishes during the weekend, which you can easily warm up or take out of the freezer during the week. Paleo bread cooked on Sundays can provide breakfast for five days. You can even prepare your egg, meat and vegetable dishes the night before.

4. *Do not be too strict about dairy*

The consumption of dairy products is controversial. Our ancestors had no milking cows at their disposal. The other disadvantage of milk is that it is processed food. The benefits of milk for health are however proven. So do not be too strict and allow yourself to drink milk. It is better to opt for whole milk, which is less processed than skimmed milk and semi-skimmed milk.

- Nutrient Deficiency? Remove it

The Paleo diet has many health benefits, but between breakfast and two other meals of the day, it is possible to miss certain nutrients. Here are nutrients at risk of deficiency:
- Vitamin D
- Iodine (present in table salt)
- Magnesium
- **Vitamin K2**

You can solve this problem by adjusting your diet or taking supplements. Pay special attention to essential nutrients. It is better to observe the paleo diet with more flexibility than to risk one's health.

Chapter Ten

Day to Day Paleo Diet Recipes

The Paleolithic Diet is a diet that has been much talked about in recent years. It allows you to lose weight and keep the line without counting calories or eating less. But many criticize it, stressing that it can be dangerous to health.

It is based on a simple idea: we are programmed to be beautiful, strong and healthy. Our genes allow it. If we get fat, get sick and have little energy, the fault is what we eat. To have a sculpted physique, therefore, it would be enough to put on the table the foods that activate the "fat burning genes." What are these foods? Those who come from Prehistory!

Diseases unknown in antiquity, such as obesity, diabetes and celiac disease (gluten intolerance, a protein complex found in cereals), would, in fact, be born together with modern nutrition, which introduced dairy products and high-index carbohydrates into the diet glycemic. By eating as we used to do millions of years ago, we could lose weight, slow down aging, lower bad cholesterol and reduce appetite.

The paleo diet is an easy type of diet to follow because it does not include calorie counting. You can eat as much as you want and strengthen your muscles by losing weight. Just take an example from what our ancestors ate. For millions of years - before the advent of agriculture - the cave dwellers only ate meat, fish, fruit, and vegetables. Nothing too elaborate! If you want to follow this diet, you have to say goodbye to refined foods and flours like pasta, cereals, sweets and sweetened carbonated drinks and instead introduce olive or coconut oil and flax seeds! Like all diets. However, should be addressed in the correct way and before trying, it is advisable that you ask your family doctor for advice to understand if there may be contraindications.

The Paleo diet, also known as a digestive diet, focuses on food intake that a typical hunter's collection would have eaten. This means meat, eggs, fish, nuts, and algae, avoiding sugar, cereals and dairy products. Any diet plan involves inevitable boredom, a monotonous "same meal, different days" that makes the wagon easy to fall. But to keep you updated, we've developed a delicious seven-day meal plan - you can strictly follow it or just think about it.

Eggs, lean meat, vegetables, and nuts, which every self-respecting cave would have died, are ideal for eating healthy and offering an excellent alternative to processed foods such as cereals, salami, ready meals, and biscuits. The plan will help you lose weight, give you an extra protein stroke on a training day or give you a tasty recipe when you eat.

Monday
- Breakfast: Sausage Omelet (72 cal). Use coconut oil (826 cal) and 2-3 large eggs to cook (220 cal). Add two roasted turkey sausages (80 cal) and a handful of green vegetables (23 cal).
- Snack: Full of almonds (576 cal)
- Lunch: Paleo lunch pack. 1 banana (105 cal), 1 apple (95 cal), 1 chicken (239 cal), hazelnuts (628 cal), 2 boiled eggs (156 cal), 200 g green pepper (40 cal)
- Snack: Chips of baked courgette (49 cal), cut into a thin squash. Install slices on a paper towel and remove excess water. Let's sit for 20 minutes. The bowl is mixed with 5ml coconut oil salt (40 cal), pepper (40 cal) and courgette slices (52 cal). Place in an oiled pan and bake at 110 ° C for 2.5 hours or until it is crisp.
- **Dinner: Spaghetti squash (31 cal)**

Tuesday
- Breakfast: Egg Cake (115 cal). Combine 12 eggs (936 cal) with 450 g of peanut sausage and 2 small onions (56 cal), 1/2 green pepper (20 cal) and as many mushrooms (22 cal) as you want. Tilt in a container and bake for 30 minutes at 175 ° C. Cool the residue.

- Snack: Beef (250 cal)
- Lunch: Avocado (160 cal) salad with tomato (17.69 cal), and add baby spinach leaves (23.18 cal) and tomatoes.
- Snack: Apple (95 cal) and 1 tbsp almond butter (614 cal)
- **Dinner: Tomato and artichoke chicken**

Wednesday

- Breakfast: Almonds (576 cal) and berries (57 cal) with coconut milk (230 cal). (Tip: Buy frozen berries to save costs.)
- Snack: Large banana (89 cal) with 1 tbsp almond butter
- Lunch: Paleo super salad (152 cal). Tilt a large number of small spinach leaves with a small handful of walnuts (654 cal), 10-12 strawberries (48 cal) (sliced), two boiled eggs and soft vinegar (18 cal).
- Snack: Full of almonds (576 cal)
- **Dinner: Chicken (239 cal), mushrooms (22 cal) and cauliflower puree (25 cal)**

Thursday

- Breakfast: Pepper (40 cal)-baked eggs (90 cal) with turkey bacon (382 cal). Heat some coconut oil (862 cal) and bake two eggs inside the pepper rings. Serve with two slices of Turkish bacon.
- Snack: Carrot sticks (41.35 cal) with guacamole (155 cal)
- Lunch: Whitefish wraps (172 cal). Grilled white fish fillets (cod, Pollak, hake). Put it in the surrounding salad (152 cal), add ½ avocado (sliced) and rub with lime (30 cal) and coriander (23 cal).
- Snack: Smoked salmon (208 cal) on slices of cucumber (15.54 cal)
- **Dinner: Tomato and artichoke chicken residues**

Friday

- Breakfast: Scrambled eggs (148 cal)
- Snack: A small number of grapes (67 cal)
- Lunch: Hot Chicken (76 cal) and Courgette Salad (66 cal)

- Snack: Beef (250 cal)
- **Dinner: Spaghetti squash (31 cal) left over**

Saturday
- Breakfast: Catching Turkish sausage (400 cal). Peel 60g turkey sausage, 1 sweet potato (86 cal) and 90g brussel idiot into pieces. Pull it all 3 eggs (75 cal) until the sausages (301 cal) are all cooked.
- Snack: Banana (89 cal)
- Lunch: Chicken salad fajitas (48 cal)
- Snack: Full of almonds (576 cal)
- **Dinner: Chicken (239 cal), mushrooms and cauliflower puree**

Sunday
- Breakfast: Scrambled eggs (148 cal)
- Snack: Banana (89 cal), blueberries (57 cal), pineapple (50 cal) and cinnamon smoothies (247 cal). Mix half of the banana, a handful of frozen blueberries, half frozen pineapple, a handful of cabbage (25 cal), 1 tbsp of almond butter and 200 ml of water in a blender.
- Lunch: Tomato and artichoke chicken residue
- Snack: Cucumbers (15.54 cal)
- **Dinner: Garlic (148.9 cal) and herb pork(100 cal) minced meat (332 cal) with dessert potato (190 cal).**

In line with this, many diseases and pathologies of the modern era were almost non-existent in the Paleolithic. Men hunted, and women gathered the fruits of nature. Everything came from nature without cultivation or intensive farming. Today modern man is overweight and out of shape, while our ancestor was more muscular and had a lower percentage of body fat. Why not try a return to the origins? According to the paleo diet cereals - for example - are not well assimilated by our body, since we are not made to take them. Most contain - indeed - gluten and lectins, to which many people are intolerant. Less consumption of refined and industrial foods - promises a paleo diet - will lower diabetes, celiac disease, and high cholesterol!

Chapter Eleven

Salt and the Paleo Diet

Salt consumption, such as carbohydrates, protein and fat, is surrounded by controversy and conflicting opinions from the medical community. The medical community generally believes that salt intake leads to high blood pressure and increases the chances of getting heart disease.

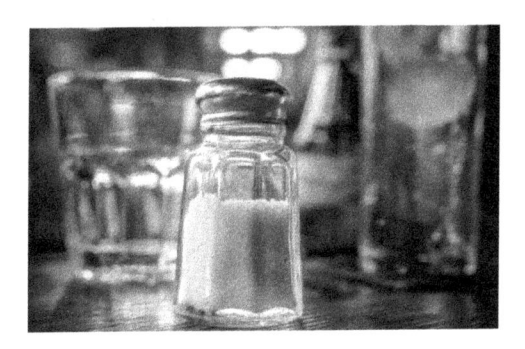

Indeed, there are a plethora of studies to suggest that this is true, especially for people who eat exclusively with industrial products. On the other hand, most research on salt consumption is done on refined and fluorinated salt, not natural, unprocessed sea salts.
The strict Paleo diet excludes salt but is it not a mistake for our health not to consume quality natural salt in the Paleo diet?
Salt is a compound of sodium and chloride. Both are electrolytes that regulate extracellular fluid volume and play a role in muscle and nerve function.
Let's look at the effects of a salt intake adapted especially during Paleo diets that promote natural foods and exclude the cooked dishes that are often too salty to enhance their taste.

The accumulation of scientific evidence shows that a low-salt diet can actually lead to severe health implications and higher overall mortality, especially in conditions such as heart disease and diabetes.

A study published in the New England Journal of Medicine with a population that consumed a moderate amount of sodium of between 3,000 and 6,000 mg/day was in better health than those who consumed either more or less than 3,000 to 6,000 mg/day. A conclusion that supports the beneficial effects of moderate sodium consumption on health.

Another study has shown that salt restriction is associated with insulin resistance, elevated triglycerides, and elevated stress hormones. Cardiac surgeon Richard Pooley does not restrict the salt or saturated fat consumption of his cardiac patients because he has not detected salt-related factors as causes of their problems.

- Medical Dangers of Too Much Sodium

Salt has a fascinating history; in the past, it was sometimes used as a currency or a reason to start a war. It is simply a natural component of seawater, left by evaporated water. Salt in the diet provides the body with the right sodium intake, which is essential for life. Although the excess of this can cause a serious imbalance in your body, increasing the risk for several potential serious medical problems.

- Sodium / Salt

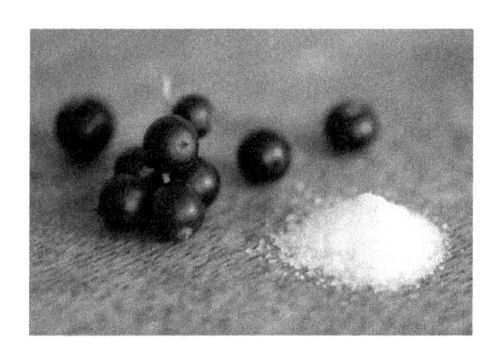

Chemically, table salt is sodium chloride, a crystalline compound that contains 40% sodium. Sodium is also a natural component found in many common foods. Our nerves use sodium to produce impulses and to contract muscles. Since sodium retains water, the body also uses it to regulate the amount of fluid in the blood, organs, and tissues. When the body contains too much sodium, the kidneys produce more urine to expel it. However, if you consume large amounts of sodium, your kidneys may not be able to handle all the excesses, risking to keep too much sodium in your body. This can cause several problems that increase the risk of serious diseases.

- High Blood Pressure

Blood pressure is an indicator of how much pressure the blood uses to radiate artery walls, heart rate and the times when the heart is "relaxed." The amount of blood in your circulation is called "blood volume," and is an important factor that determines blood pressure. When more salt is eaten than the kidneys can handle, excess salt retains water and increases the "blood volume," increasing blood pressure. High blood pressure can cause serious health problems, especially because it does not produce early symptoms.

- Heart Disease and Stroke

When too much sodium is consumed and the blood pressure is too high, over time, the extra pressure can make the vessels less elastic and more susceptible to the accumulation of fatty deposits called plaques. The health consequences of these include atherosclerosis or hardening of the arteries. In atherosclerosis, the vessels tighten, and their walls thicken, creating extra work for the heart and increasing the risk of heart attack, heart attack, and stroke. According to the Harvard School of Public Health, increased salt intake can cause a 23% increase in the aforementioned diseases and increase heart disease by 14%.

- Other Issues

According to Harvard experts, those who consume too much salt can have osteoporosis, or thinning of the bones, as salt abuse tends to wear down calcium from the bones. High sodium intake can also increase the risk of developing stomach cancer, according to the World Cancer Research Fund and the American Institute for Cancer Research.

- Lowering Salt Intake

The National Heart, Lung and Blood Institute recommends that healthy adults consume no more than 2,400 milligrams of sodium per day, equivalent to 6 grams of table salt or about 1 teaspoon. If you have or are at risk of high blood pressure, it is recommended to consume only 1,500 milligrams a day. Use less salt at the table or replace it with herbs and spices without salt, and check the seasoning labels for the amount of salt content. Choose fresh fruits and vegetables and rinse salads and canned vegetables before serving. Choose low-salt products and check the wording for "hidden" salt on product labels, avoiding sodium bicarbonate, sodium nitrate, sodium citrate, and sodium benzoate.

Tips for Consuming Salt in The Paleo Diet Reasonably

To consume salt in the Paleo diet in a reasonable way here are the 7 points to respect:

- Use natural and unrefined sea salt. Pollution of the seas and oceans around the world means that some salts may contain mercury and other toxic heavy metals.

- Always salted your food after tasting it to avoid adding too much salt.
- If you have a Paleo diet based on mostly raw organic products, quality meats with outdoor animals and seafood using quality salt this will enhance the taste and cover your body's salt needs.
- If you drink enough water, adding a pinch of quality sea salt to every liter of water you drink will help maintain electrolyte levels and optimal energy levels.
- If you generously salty your food or eat processed foods, your water needs to be reduced or not salted as this can actually cause more harm than good and have adverse effects on your health.
- **Athletes who experience a significant loss of electrolyte through perspiration, with the use of quality sea salt on their food and in water avoid this deficit of electrolytes and maintain high energy levels.**

Balance disorders, head turning (due to low blood pressure) is a symptom related to low level of electrolyte. This can often be avoided by following the guidelines below.

The Paleo diet is naturally diuretic by the high consumption of vegetables, and it is essential to have a supply of water and sufficient salt.

If you suffer from weakness, constipation, fatigue, cramps, headaches, head turning when you get up, add natural salt, without additives, non-fluorinated, unrefined to your water and your diet. You can also supplement electrolytes or drink bone broths to avoid these inconveniences.

In summary, ban refined salt from your diet and promote moderate consumption of natural sea salt or quality salt flower as part of a Paleo food style.

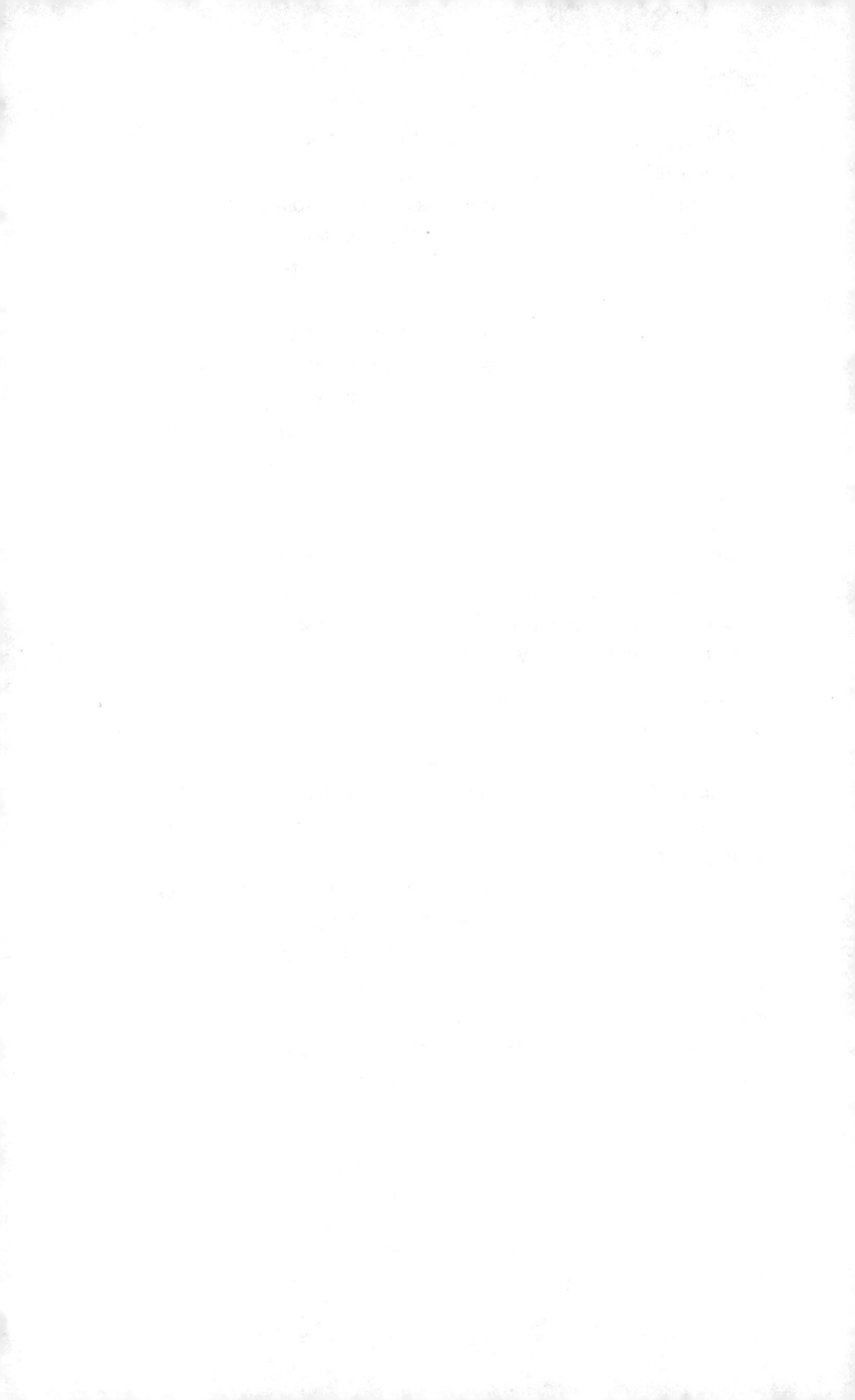